THE
GENTLEMAN'S
GUIDE TO
COOL

clothing, grooming, etiquette

PAUL GILES

JoJo
PUBLISHING

THE GENTLEMAN'S GUIDE TO COOL:
Clothing, Grooming, Etiquette
Paul Giles

Published by Classic Author and Publishing Services Pty Ltd.
Imprint of JoJo Publishing.
First published 2015

'Yarra's Edge'
2203/80 Lorimer Street
Docklands VIC 3008
Australia

Email: admin@classic-jojo.com or visit www.classic-jojo.com

JoJo Publishing

Editor: Julie Athanasiou
Designer / typesetter: Working Type Studio (www.workingtype.com.au)
Printed in China by Ink Asia.

National Library of Australia Cataloguing-in-Publication entry

Creator: Giles, Paul Antony, author.
Title: The Gentleman's Guide to Cool : clothing, grooming & etiquette / Paul Giles.
ISBN: 9780994183828 (paperback)
Subjects: Men's clothing.
             Grooming for men.
             Fashion--Social aspects.
Dewey Number: 391.1

This book is dedicated to my mum and brothers,
who raised me and guided me toward a privileged life.

CONTENTS

My Story

....

I grew up in the 1970s in East Bentleigh, then a tough working class suburb of Melbourne about 18 kilometres south east of the central business district. The men around me all made their living in factories, on building sites or working for the Government. The standard uniform for both work and play in East Bentleigh was flannelette shirts, blue singlets and Hard Yakka pants. From an early age it was instilled in me that being a man and being interested in fashion were completely contradictory. Attending secondary school at Moorabbin Tech meant having dirt under our nails, greasy hair and battle scars from school fights. Any interest in clothing, let alone any grooming routine consisting of more than velvet soap and a cut-throat razor, was seen as sissy.

By my late teens, obsessed with girls and going out on Friday nights, I quickly learned that the time I spent on my appearance through clothing and grooming practices brought great rewards. I began to observe guys from different suburbs who took the time and effort in their appearance. The clothes they wore were different; their hairstyles crafted and styled, things never seen in our neighborhood. Even the shops in their part of town were different; clothing stores and window displays with mannequins wearing colorful, tailored and modern attire. I remember riding my bike to these shops and discreetly looking from every angle and viewpoint for hours. In these parts of town the guys would wear a lemon-coloured jumper with a baby blue-coloured shirt coupled with green cords. Girls admired their every move. These guys weren't called 'poofters' for looking good and I wanted to be like them. I would happily catch the train into the city and walk for hours to look at the stores and see what was 'in' and how outfits were put together. I would scour over every advertising campaign on route and soak up as much visual information about men's fashion as possible.

As my interest in fashion grew, I observed people in movies, music videos and magazines with great attention. I noticed men of status, respect and popularity paid attention to their clothing, appearance and physique. The movie *Top Gun* exposed me to leather bomber jackets and aviator sunglasses — two items I still wear today. *An Officer and a Gentleman* showed me how to be cool and comfortable around girls and to treat them with old-fashioned values and respect. In music, Wham! showed me how styled hair, polished white teeth and a suntan could also be a male thing. Duran Duran taught me how to experiment with clothing for more formal events like weddings. On TV, *Happy Days* revealed the American Ivy League College-look, which has had a lasting influence on me, while *Miami Vice* exposed me to quality Italian tailoring, smart summer dressing, pastel colours, linen, loafers and no socks. Looking back, these movies and TV shows had a huge impact on my development throughout my teenage years and beyond.

Added to these influences were my two older brothers, who were both building careers in AFL. By following them around the football grounds I went from my local neighborhood to new areas way across town, which brought new people, places, styles and ideas into my life. When my brothers started to get well paid in their football careers, they started to experiment with clothes as well. Like any younger brother I secretly tried on the shirts and jackets they brought home, desperately looking forward to the day my body would fill out and the clothes would fit properly so I could borrow them. Hanging out around men five to ten years older than me turned out to be a brilliant learning curve. I realised by having the confidence to create their own individual style and to separate themselves from the rest of the pack, these men earned respect and popularity not only from their peers, but more importantly to me, from women.

In 1987 I was out of high school and working for the Moorabbin City Council. During the colder months I was a gardener and during the summer months I worked as a lifeguard at Moorabbin pool. When a mate suggested I visit a modelling agency, I thought he was crazy. I guess the by-product of working as a lifeguard was a suntan, fit physique and healthy appearance.

To my great surprise, within two weeks of my first interview I was on a plane bound for Tokyo. I'd swapped my swimming shorts for jeans, aviator sunglasses, white T-shirt and linen jacket — a Tom Cruise meets Don Johnson meets Fonzie sort of look. It was quite a contrast sitting poolside one week to working in a city of 10 million people the next.

As a new model I had to show up at eight to ten job castings every day. Like at any job interview I had to show the client why I was the best candidate, which involved showing my portfolio of photos, trying on clothes and acting out the role required for the advertising campaign. Look happy and cool. Look rich and successful. Look mature and in love. Look funky, athletic, adventurous, and energetic. My success depended on how well I presented myself, how I carried myself and how good I looked. I must have been doing something right because in my first week I landed a magazine cover that changed my life. *TARZAN* had a circulation of five million readers. Its previous cover identities included sports stars Carl Lewis and Mike Tyson, and actor Mickey Rourke. Over the course of several months I stayed in Tokyo, working for designers such as Yohji Yamamoto and Issey Miyake, where I learnt the importance of clothing fit, colour and style.

A year later I moved to the US, commuting between Los Angeles, Chicago and New York to work with gilt-edged clients including Calvin Klein, Ralph Lauren, GAP, Nike, DKNY and Hugo Boss. I was featured in catalogues, television commercials and on billboards. Whilst working amongst the best designers, photographers and stylists, I observed and learnt the importance of aesthetics and how colours, textures and patterns could be mixed, matched and incorporated into a complete look. I observed how experts in their craft combined these to create clothing outfits, props, backdrops, settings and moods to create fascinating billboards, magazine advertisements and television commercials. I was getting paid to observe and learn what could not be learned through text books.

Over the next four years I commuted between the US and Tokyo before returning briefly to Australia for SABA, Sportscraft and Adidas campaigns. After that I focused on magazine and television work in Europe, the US, Japan and New Zealand. Eventually relocating to Sydney, I worked with David Jones, Myer, Country Road, Marcs and Morrissey, and had a regular contract with a television games show before starting my own family and changing direction.

How I can help you

"With confidence, you have won before you have started."
— **Marcus Garvey**

At 5 feet 10 inches tall with hair like wire I was not the stereotypical male model measurements and attributes needed to succeed in an industry based on appearance. To come up against men in job castings who were from European backgrounds, who had the perfect dimensions, chiselled features, dark skin, thick hair and athlete physiques should have been intimidating and embarrassing.

But I was never overawed or discouraged as I had the self-knowledge to overcome my personal flaws, and this gave me the confidence to compete successfully in an extremely competitive industry. I learnt how to present myself so I looked taller, fitter and healthier than my counterparts. I got job after job and enjoyed a global career lasting two decades.

Knowing you have fully given something your absolute best will allow you to have the confidence to do anything. I have witnessed firsthand how if you present yourself to the best of your ability your mind set changes, your appeal broadens, and good things start to happen in your life.

In today's world it is almost expected that men be successful, strong, positive, healthy and confident. A perfectly run machine with the answers to all of life's hiccups, the wisdom to look after the future and provide an idyllic and serene environment, all while being admired and respected by family and peers. In a perfect world this is how we would all like to live our lives, and I'm here to tell you guys that we can. The best and easiest way to begin this process is to know yourself and present yourself accordingly to the world.

Women have lots of information available to them about how to dress, how to look after their skin, and matters of etiquette, but it seems to me there's not much around for men. I think it's just as important men have the same opportunity to learn how to project the best possible side of themselves. Today's technology makes it too easy for us guys to be compared and judged against men from a breadth of categories, fields, occupations and lifestyles. With these comparisons it is easy to feel inadequate and insecure. We know it's the person inside that matters most, but like it or not we are judged first on the outside. One has to be lured to the door before it can be opened and explored on the inside. On those occasions when you do wear a suit or dress more upmarket, haven't you noticed the difference in the way you are seen and treated compared to when you wear trackies and ugg boots?

Your image is the perception people take from your appearance, manners, etiquette and posture. According to one Harvard University study, 55 per cent of a woman's opinion about you is based on the way you look the first time she meets you. You never get a second chance to make a first impression.

The information I have put together in this book has been accumulated over many years of practical experience. With a few simple skills and knowledge of how the right clothes, accessories, routines and practices can enhance your image and personal style, you will have the confidence to achieve anything you desire. We all have a body with two arms and two legs, so why not make the most of them and wear the correct clothes to be the best man you can. It's easy.

In this book I share with you the tools to create an image that reflects your personality and style, and enhances your confidence. A first impression of a man who's classy, elegant, courteous and fun to be around is something that's in your power to build yourself. Using this book you can put together a versatile, practical and effective wardrobe, learn to coordinate your clothes, dress for any occasion and learn some simple grooming techniques.

To reach the top the first steps are often the hardest, but the confidence ladder is worth the climb.

Chapter 1:
Know Yourself First

Your way, not the highway:
How to develop your own style

It still amazes me every time I go shopping that I see a large percentage of women select and decide what their man should or should not wear. Far too many men have gone through life having their style dictated to them by their mothers, then by their girlfriends, and then their wives.

If you've never taken a shot at creating your own style, a good time to start is now. The most important aspect of developing your own style is remaining true to yourself. There are enough styles out there to make everyone comfortable in developing their own, no matter what age, size, demographic or situation.

To help define your own style, a good reference point is to take a look at public figures from the music, movie, sport and television industries. Observe what makes them stylish, individual and cool. In particular, check out what and how they wear clothing and accessories, what hairstyle they wear, how they dress for the occasion and how they conduct themselves as a whole. I began this process as a teenager, and today still observe with great interest what is going on.

Television, magazines, catalogues and the internet provide

a plethora of images and information, but please draw the line somewhere, as these folk like to draw attention to themselves. You don't have to emulate them completely, just observe to gain ideas and starting points. Take one thing you like from five different references, put it all together and create your own individual style.

Here are my tips for creating your own style:
- Be yourself and feel comfortable. Wear what you think looks good, not what others think looks good.
- You should always feel comfortable with what you're wearing, so stay with items that suit your personality and style, while keeping the occasion and setting in mind.
- The key to individual style is always to match it to your personality, age and personal features.
- Don't overdo it or think expensive clothes are the only answer for style.
- Have a go! You've got nothing to lose and will be more confident for the experience.

It takes all shapes & sizes:
Dressing for your body shape

When buying clothes, the paramount rule to remember is to buy garments suitable for your body shape. No matter how expensive the clothes, if the fit is not right, not only have you wasted your money, but you may be exacerbating what you are actually trying to hide.

Fit, cut and colour are the three ingredients to help you choose your wardrobe — it doesn't matter if you are large, skinny, short or tall, the following basic rules will help guide you towards a better understanding for your next purchase.

Large men

Big men should stay away from baggy clothes because they add weight and size to your frame. Wear dark colours like black, navy, brown and grey, and avoid horizontal and diagonal stripes. Vertical patterns and pinstripes will elongate your silhouette. Wear relaxed-fit trousers and single-breasted jackets. Stay clear of turtlenecks and opt for V-neck jumpers and T-shirts instead.

Thin men

Skinny guys should avoid very tight-fitted clothes and head-to-toe solid dark colours. Whites, creams and pastels will give the impression of bulk for upper body, and a contrast between dark pants and a light top will break up the beanpole look. Choose horizontal stripe patterns instead of vertical lines to give the impression of broadness. A double-breasted jacket will also add width.

Short men

Men lacking height should steer clear of stark colour contrasts between the top and bottom half, and choose colours from the same family to give a fluid, elongated impression. This is easy enough when you wear a suit, since the jacket and pants are made to match. For more casual wear, choose blue denim jeans with a dark blue top, and khaki shorts with neutral earthy colours on top. Choose a key colour and mix it with slight variations of that hue.

Also stay away from large prints and opt for thin vertical stripes instead. Avoid heavy twill fabric for jackets and ensure pants are tailored with a plain hem and no cuff or tapering. I followed these tips throughout my career and looked and, more importantly, felt two inches taller.

Tall men

If you're tall you should exclude both oversized and tight-fitting clothing, as either way will give the impression of having awkward and gangly limbs. Contrasting colours will help break up your long line, so pair different coloured shirts and pants. Wearing straight-legged trousers and jeans coupled with wide belts, and double-breasted jackets with wide ties, will help balance proportions.

True colours shining through: Choosing the right colours

Wearing the right colours will make you look healthier. It will not only help make your skin glow, but also bring your features to life. On the flipside, the wrong colours can make you look drab or washed out.

Here are a few general guidelines to help you determine which colours best match your features and skin tone. Men with dark skin, brown hair and brown eyes look best in bright colours and different shades of white, due to the contrast. Sapphire blue, ruby red and bold colours such as orange and green are also good choices.

Men with an olive to medium-toned skin tone, blue, green or hazel eyes, and medium to light hair should choose earthy tones such as brown, olive green, camel and ivory.

Men with light features should choose cooler colours such as grey, pale and navy blue, green and khaki.

To play it safe use the above colour methodology in the cooler months for items such as shirts, V-neck jumpers, scarves and beanies. Only a small amount of your ideal colour tone is required to bring out your features and enhance your skin tone.

Regardless of your skin type, eye and hair colour, keep in mind that you can rarely go wrong with basic colours such as black, grey, navy blue, brown and most earthy tones. These solid, dependable colours are perfect for outer layers such as coats, jackets, pants and knits. Choosing classic colours is a good idea style-wise, as they are easy to mix and match, and their timeless nature makes them the practical choice, long-lasting and promises value for money.

During the warm weather, blue skies and sun-baked skin lend themselves to experimenting with styles and including more colour. A breadth of colours are available in all types of T-shirts. Crew neck and V-neck are good options for the under 30-year-olds, with polo shirts the pick for all age groups. The polo shirt comes in an array of colours for all skin types and gives a more dressed-up look.

Shorts come in an assortment of colours, styles and patterns. The board short offers every print and pattern imaginable, so choose wisely. One bold piece of coloured clothing can be eye-catching and very noticeable, but more than one and you run the risk of looking like a neon casino sign. If you choose to wear colourful shorts, put on a plain shirt to go with it. And if you're in the mood for a colourful shirt, pair it with plain shorts.

To incorporate a little fun, individuality and colour to your attire, consider coloured belts, watch bands, thongs (flip flops) and sunglasses.

Act your age, not your shoe size: Dressing your age

Dress for your age. Not the age you wish you still were. Not the age you'll one day become. No matter what brand of clothing or how expensive it might be, a 50-year-old man dressing like a 20-year-old and vice versa is without doubt the biggest individual fashion mistake any man can make.

Twenties

Men in their twenties often haven't figured out their own style yet — they tend to dress like their mates to fit in. You are in your prime in regards to physique and supple skin so experiment but ensure you get clothes that fit.

Lose the logos and invest in some quality pieces to see you through, like a tailored blazer and a good quality dress shirt. That special person in your life will appreciate your individuality and creativity, plus you will stand out from your mates.

Twenties style icons

There are currently plenty of 'style icons' in their twenties you can look to for ideas on classic, individual dressing. For example, Zac Efron progressed from the teeny bopper image of wearing baggy, ill-fitted jeans, runners and waistcoats to a stylish, gentlemanly way of dressing. Wearing clothing that fit his body correctly changed everything.

English rapper Tinie Tempah is an example of someone who has the perfect eye in mixing classic tailoring with a sports edge to create his own style, and he has a great eye for detail. He starts with the bottom half by combining dark-wash denim and retro influenced footwear and builds the top with tailored layers such as vests, patterned shirts, slim-lined blazers and bow ties.

Thirties

Once you hit 30, it is time to develop your signature style and to dress well for all occasions, both work and social. Avoid items that will draw attention and make you stand out from the crowd, such as slogan T-shirts, sporting team colours or fluorescent and shinny sportswear.

To advance your career, purchase quality over quantity. Move away from the high-top sneakers, shabby jeans and surf attire. If you dress casually, be prepared to be treated casually. Dark straight-leg jeans, chinos, polo shirts and loafers will give a well-groomed professional look without trying too hard. The best investment is a bespoke (individually patterned and crafted) tailored suit.

Thirties style icons

David Beckham is the most influential man on the planet when it comes to all things style. He is a continuing and evolving trendsetter showing the way with a perfect balance between formal, business and casual wear. He continually stays on top of trends, and creates his own by wearing items out of context and breaking all the style rules. He has now found the perfect balance of being stylish without being too metrosexual in his dress.

Ryan Gosling is a great model for change, progressing from awkwardly fitted suits and teenage graphic tees to sleek, precise tailoring and a cool casual style with his own twist. He compliments his slim, athletic build by keeping the accessories to a minimum. He is simplistic and minimalist in both his casual and formal looks.

Forties

Men in their forties have to find a balance between dressing too young and dressing too old. If you tip the scales either way it could give off the dreaded impression of a mid-life crisis! The most important thing to remember is to look for reputable brands in simple colours, with a good cut that flatters your body shape. Choose quality materials and don't over-accessorise. It is better to have 12 versatile quality items than 30 trendy pieces. A watch is a great investment piece.

Forties style icons

Daniel Craig always looks comfortable and classic without losing his masculinity or individuality. He realised the importance of clothing fit once he reached the age of 30, evolving from an oversized jacket and pleat trousers to a sleek and trim-fitting stylish 40-year-old.

Brad Pitt has a natural ability in regards to dress-sense, and has never tried too hard, whether he is in a three-piece suit or casually riding his motorbike. His fashion choices are refreshingly down-to-earth, as he stays within a neutral palette and dark hues and avoids ostentatious printed pieces.

Fifties

Once you hit the big five-O, nothing less than very smart-casual is acceptable, remembering less is more, plain is good and quality is the key. Dress for your body shape, ensuring a perfect fit. Avoid bright primary colours and stay with dark and earthy hues instead. Also avoid sneakers, obvious gold chains and Speedos. A high-quality, tailored trench coat is your best investment.

Fifties style icons

George Clooney, admired by men and women alike, always wears investment quality pieces, and made not wearing a tie cool. He wears the basics without all the bells and whistles by combining tailored black suits for formal events, and gray chinos with white T-shirts for his downtime. He also made the no-fuss clothing and hairstyles cool, is happy being 50 years young and it shows.

Steve McQueen gave the all-American look a rugged edge by way of sunglasses, slim-cut tailored suits, sport coats, zip-up windbreakers, chinos, V-neck jumpers, shawl-collared cardigans and polo shirts. He was the 'King of Cool' for a reason.

When size does matter: Knowing your exact measurements

Knowing your exact clothing measurements is one of the most valuable pieces of information for saving you time and money. Whether shopping online, browsing the sale rack or placing orders with friends who are heading overseas, knowing this simple information is invaluable.

The following instructions describe how to measure yourself correctly — that's using a clothing measuring tape, not a building measuring tape, guys — and in turn, determining your correct sizing for both clothing and footwear.

1. Chest

Wrap the tape measure under your armpits and around the bulkiest part of your chest and shoulder blades without flexing.

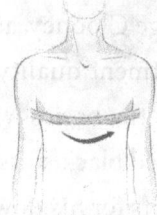

2. Neck

Measure around the base of your neck, a few centimetres below your Adam's apple. To ensure extra comfort and room, slip two fingers inside the tape — this will give the shirt a natural look if your top button is done up.

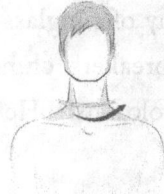

3. Sleeve

Hold your arm straight out from your side and ask someone to measure from your shoulder joint to your wrist joint.

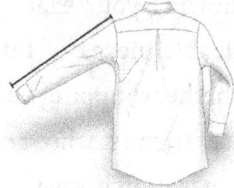

4. Waist

Wrap the tape measure around your torso where you would normally wear a belt, approximately four centimetres below your navel. Don't pull the tape too tight — you should be able to place a finger between your body and the tape.

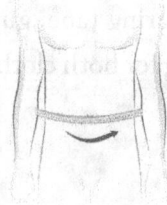

5. Inseam

To get an exact measurement this is achieved more easily with two people. Very carefully, place the top of the tape where your leg begins up near the 'family jewels' region and measure down to the ankle bone.

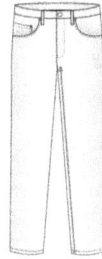

6. Outer seam

Hold the tape at the top of your waistband on the outside of your leg and have someone measure the distance to the bottom of your ankle, or where you like your pants to end.

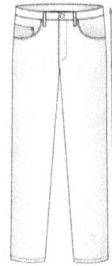

7. Foot

Whilst wearing socks, place the tape on the ground and stand on it. Allow an extra thumb-width from your big toe to the end of the shoe for correct fit and comfort.

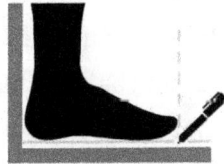

Measure and record in both centimetres and inches, as USA, Asian and European sizing are in different formats. If your weight fluctuates, it would be best to take the time to measure yourself before every shopping adventure. Take the time to know this information, as correct fit is the key to looking your best.

Just goin' to the shop: Key shopping tips

For most men, shopping for clothes can be a painful experience. The thought of trying on numerous items of clothing for a new set of threads sounds like a chore to most guys, who shop only out of pure necessity. With time a commodity, a few simple tips will have you in and out in no time, and looking a million bucks.

Before you even hit the shops, scanning the latest fashion magazines and websites to find out what's in style each season will give you a clearer picture of what you may require. Take note of styles, colours and fabrics, as this will reduce aimless window shopping time. Knowing your measurements will help speed up the process because you'll be able to pick out garments faster, and you'll also be more likely to choose articles that fit right the first time, reducing time in the fitting room.

Pick your time and place to go shopping. Avoid peak times, as crowds are the last thing you need. Early weekend mornings are the best time, and it's also easier to get a parking space.

Before leaving the house, make a list of the items you're planning to buy and be clear about the amount of money you want to spend. Do not enter stores or sections not on your list — this will reduce impulse buys.

When entering a store, try to locate the items you need and don't allow yourself to become overwhelmed by racks and shelves full of merchandise. Stay true to your list and don't waver from the colour, pattern, fabric or style. Be decisive and ask sales assistants if they have what you need in stock or if they can order it in.

Wear clothes on your shopping trip that are practical and easy to change in and out of, such as a T-shirt, zip-up sweater and slip on shoes, instead of buttoned shirts and lace-up boots. This will minimise your fitting room blues.

Sales are the perfect time to build your wardrobe for a fraction of the price.

Here are a few ways to save you time, money and disappointment:

Know your sizing and do your research. Knowing your measurements will save you a lot of pain. Search the store online first, or call to ensure they have what you are looking for and if the price has been discounted.

Buy quality not quantity. This is the time when high-end brands and products are more affordable. Purchase investment pieces that are not trend-based, but timeless and of high craftsmanship instead.

Make a list and set a budget. Do not impulse buy or overspend, stay true to your list.

Ask yourself if you would buy it at full price. Do not be lured to buying stuff because it is cheap, unless it is the necessities of socks and jocks.

Will you like the item this time next year? Stay away from fads in the way of patterns and seasonal colours.

Wear comfortable clothing such as drawstring pants, clothing with zips instead of buttons and slip-on shoes to make things easier when trying on clothes.

Don't rush to the checkout. If you are uncertain about the item, hold on to it whilst roaming around the store. Putting it back on the rack may lead to disappointment.

Online shopping

Online shopping has its advantages, but requires a degree of caution. There is always the chance you will be disappointed with the quality, fit or colour. By following these tips, you'll be able to easily find reputable retailers and have the luxury of buying speciality items not yet available in Australian stores.

Here are my tips for online shopping:

- **Know your size**

  Know exactly what size, style and fit of clothes you are looking for. Measure your waist, chest, hips, inseam and arm length as explained earlier in the chapter. By doing this you will minimise the stress of exchange and refunds.

- **Research and analyse your seller**

  Search for websites that offer extensive information about the products they offer. The best, most reputable websites will include in-depth sizing information, detailed descriptions of each product and high quality pictures of every clothing item offered.

- **Check your shipping/mailing rate**

  One of the biggest complaints online shoppers have is the high cost of shipping. Ensure you carefully read the cost details according to the size and weight of what you are buying.

- **Read the FAQs and fine print**

  Most professional sites will offer a listing of FAQs (frequently asked questions). These questions should answer basic concerns about shipping rates, return policies and payment security. All reputable merchants have secure sites that protect the security of your credit card and personal information. Look carefully for any fine print or special terms and conditions.

Chapter 2:
Your Wardrobe Essentials

Wardrobe DNA: The 12 essential wardrobe items

A strong foundation is essential to any sound structure and your wardrobe is no exception. To create a versatile, stylish, timeless and affordable wardrobe start with these 12 basics, which will cover every occasion and lifestyle:

1. The classic single-breasted suit in a dark colour such as navy, grey or charcoal. Wear the jacket over a polo shirt or business shirt with jeans or chinos for a more casual look.
2. A white or pale blue business shirt worn with a suit or with jeans or chinos.
3. Dark blue denim straight-cut jeans paired with a business shirt, polo shirt or white crew-neck T-shirt.
4. Polo shirts in black, white or a pastel colour paired with chinos, jeans or khaki shorts with sneakers or loafers for the weekend.
5. A V-neck jumper in a dark blue or brown over a shirt paired with jeans or chinos always looks stylish.
6. Chino pants are the complete versatile essential, worn casual with a polo shirt or dressed up with a jacket.
7. Black brogues or Oxford lace-ups are the suit staple, and are good for dressing up casual jeans or chinos.

8. A white crew-neck T-shirt can be worn with jeans or shorts, or under a shirt for added warmth.

9. Khaki shorts with a polo or business shirt combined with loafers are good for the warmer months.

10. Brown leather loafers are the most versatile shoe, a timeless classic for all occasions.

11. Grey track pants and a hoodie as exercise and lounge gear is never out-dated.

12. Accessory staples include a black and a brown belt, striped tie, black beanie, Panama hat, black, navy, white and grey socks, metal-frame sunglasses and coloured (clean!) underwear.

If it suits you: Choosing the right suit

Every man should own at least one suit — and with my help it will be the perfect suit for work, weddings, funerals, parties and every type of occasion in between.

Purchasing your next suit with no thought beforehand will increase the risk of wasting lots of money and looking like a cross between Pee Wee Herman and Mr Bean, instead of the dapper, powerful and charismatic man you are. A well-fitted, stylish suit exudes class, confidence and sophistication. And women love a man in a good suit.

You have two different style options in regards to the jacket: single or double-breasted. A double-breasted jacket overlaps at the front, while a single-breasted one doesn't.

The classic, simple look of the single-breasted jacket makes it the more versatile and fashionable of the two styles and a better choice for first-time buyers. Double-breasted jackets are generally more formal; however you will see many menswear designers and retailers pairing double-breasted jackets with a pair of jeans to dress it down. Also remember that double-breasted jackets look best on long, lean physiques and can make short men look stouter.

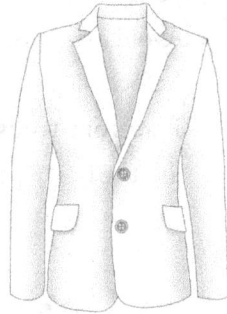

single-breasted jacket

When choosing a fabric, wool is your best option. It is the most comfortable, wrinkle-resistant and long lasting. Another plus is the fabric's ability to absorb moisture; so on those hot days when such attire is a pre-requisite, it will help keep you cooler. In regards to colour, a navy suit is the most versatile, lending itself to all manner of formal affairs. Navy is also the best colour to pair up shirts and ties. If you already have a navy suit, charcoal would be the next alternative.

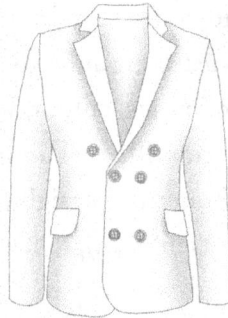

double-breasted jacket

Suit Tips

Here are my suits for buying the right suit:

- Keep it simple and classic; choose suits with three-buttons for double-breasted suits and two-buttons for a single-breasted suit.
- Keep the shoulder natural and stay away from too much padding.
- Lapels talk: a small, high-notched lapel, right on the collarbone is the mark of a good suit.

- Ensure the jacket is slightly fitted in the waist area, to give your body a more dynamic shape.
- Avoid extra pockets and fancy stitching, as it will be out-dated before the second wear.
- Flat-front trousers are more modern and classic, but pleats are the best option for larger-waisted men.

It's all in the jeans: Buying jeans

A trusty pair of denim jeans is the most essential and versatile item in your wardrobe. But buying them can be the most confusing, frustrating and agonising process for a man. The different choices in brands, cut, fit, wash, length and style are endless. And there seems like a hundred cuts from boot-cut, slim-fit, relaxed-fit, skinny and straight, in washes from raw, acid, dirty to stone.

Denim originated more than 100 years ago and was worn by prisoners as part of their uniform. Today jeans are a staple of everyone's wardrobe. Each season brings with it new trends, treatments and features. My tip is not to get seduced by the fly-by-night trends, and keep your jeans simple and basic. Ageless brands provide value for money. Buying something ripped, torn and already worn out for $500 is not my idea of a good deal .

Keep your colours basic and over time they will fade and get holes naturally, so you can be the smart and cool one for a fraction of the price. Boot and straight-cut jeans are the timeless classics for most body types. If you're thin have a go at slim and skinny jeans, while bigger blokes can try a relaxed-fit.

The most important thing to consider with jeans is the cut:

- Boot-cut: Slim-fit jeans cut with a slight flare are perfect for most body types.
- Relaxed-fit: Loose cut from the waist are perfect for the heavier man.
- Skinny: Ultra skin-tight jeans are good for the twiggy body shapes.
- Slim-fit: Tapered but not form-fitting styles suit the medium-body shape.
- Straight-cut: Classic, with a discreet straight leg, this style is suitable for most body shapes.

Jean Tips

These are my tips for buying jeans:
- Keep it simple when choosing colour, as washed trends come and go quickly.
- Stay with old-school brands like Levi's, Lee and Wrangler, as they are good value and will age well. For as long as I can remember Wrangler and Edwin have been my brands of choice.
- When going shopping, take the two pairs of shoes you will be wearing most with the jeans, so you can see what they look like when trying them on.
- Once you find the perfect pair, buy a pair each in dark blue, white, black and charcoal.
- Always wash your jeans inside out and hang to dry out of the sun to avoid fading.
- Know your size and search second-hand stores for a bargain.
- Stay clear of embroidery and large rear pockets.

Mr. T: The classic T-shirt

I can't remember a time in my life when I did not own a T-shirt, and I am sure most men are the same. I was fascinated by how someone like James Dean could look so cool wearing only jeans and a white T-shirt. As my intrigue and interest in fashion grew, I discovered his secret was the simplicity of a white crew-neck cotton T-shirt. Over my life's journey, my T-shirt wearing trends and phases have covered all sorts of styles.

Men under 25 can get away with any type of T-shirt. This includes crew-neck, V-neck and slim-fit in any colour and pattern, proudly displaying logos and designs, symbols and pictures that broadcast their favourite bands, brands, clubs and icons. This age bracket allows you to reveal and proudly display your likes and support for what and who you admire.

The 25–35 year olds should avoid comical slogans, wrestler portraits and chauvinist rap artists, and keep the sporting and surf-wear brands for the weekend attire. You look casual so be prepared to be treated the same.

Any age upwards of 40 should stay away from graphics, V-necks, button-ups and muscle shirts, and make colours and stripes the point of difference. This will show a fun side of your personality in a contemporary and gentlemanly way.

Fabrics, design, cuts, colours, shapes, logos, images and branding have all seen the T-shirt go through some changes, and I suggest we follow the changes as our age and physique change too.

No matter what age you fall into, every male should have three staple T-shirts:

1. The white cotton crew-neck goes with anything and everything. Just make sure it's 100 per cent cotton. Fitted is good, snug is a gamble and tight is just plain wrong!

2. The grey cotton ringer T-shirt features more detail around the collar and sleeves. It's perfect for the weekend and a sports necessity.

3. The stylish, reliable polo shirt. Choose one in either a bright colour (orange, yellow, green or aqua), or one that features stripes as this will portray sophistication, elegance and effort.

If you want to wear a statement, slogan or graphic T-shirt, only wear it in public if you feel comfortable in doing so in front of your mother in-law, boss and at school pick-up.

A lot of things look good with age, but T-shirts are the exception. Once underarms become yellow, the shape has been lost and stains can't be removed, it's time for 'out with the old and in with the new'. My favourite T-shirt is the white Hanes crew-neck and has been part of my attire since I was 16-years-old. Whenever anyone I knew was going overseas I would place my order for a pack of three.

Warm as toast: The coat

During the cold months of winter there is no better piece of clothing to keep the body and soul warm than the indispensable coat. The difference between a coat and jacket is that a jacket ends at the hips, while a coat ends at the middle of the thigh.

Coats in general are manufactured from a thicker fabric to add warmth, whilst jackets are designed more for looks and at times wind protection. When choosing a coat, the two most important things to consider are fabric and fit. For warmth and durability, 100 per cent wool and wool blends are by far your best option. If you're a cold fish and need a little extra warmth, opt for one that also has a thin layer of thinsulate, goose or synthetic down sewn into the lining.

To have you looking and feeling comfortable, choosing the perfectly fitted coat is paramount. The rule of thumb is to simply move up one size over your suit jacket size as this allows you to move easily without the layers binding at your shoulders and neck. The shoulder seams should fall just over the edge of your natural shoulder, hence allowing normal movement, perfect silhouette and fabric drape.

Purchasing a new winter coat will fall into one of three categories: the parka, the everyday and the formal.

Classic parka

The classic parka is best with casual wear, but can be worn with a suit briefly when needed. Just ensure it is longer than your suit jacket. This jacket will offer more versatility in a navy, charcoal or olive green. Limit the logos, chunky zippers, cords and Velcro tabs.

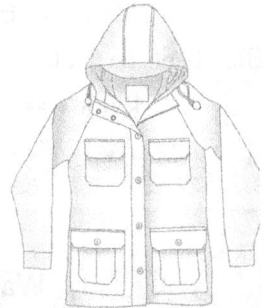

Everyday coat

The everyday coat is a multi-tasker, which can be used seven days a week. It is upmarket enough for office attire and adds style and sophistication to the weekend outfit. The duffle coat and the pea coat are timeless classics.

Duffle coat

The duffle coat gets its name from the Belgium town of Duffel where double-faced thick wool has been made for centuries, but it wasn't until the British Royal Navy opted for the uniform attire of coats manufactured from this fabric that the town became world renowned. Recognisable by its wooden toggle fasteners, it was designed for navy seamen with cold, frostbitten fingers to fasten the coat with ease. The oversized attached hood was to accommodate naval caps.

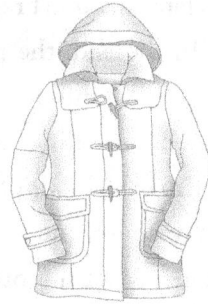

Due to its history, it teams well with stripes, navy blazers, dark jeans and chinos, beanie hats and thick cable-knit jumpers. As for colours, the duffle coat tends to look best in your timeless neutrals of navy, black, brown and grey, as it often has to deal with the cold elements. Darker tones will also hide weather stains much better. These colours will never go out of style, and will anchor or coordinate with nearly every other item you have in your wardrobe.

Pea coat

The pea coat, the double-breasted wool coat with broad lapels, has been worn since the 18th century and originated from the maritime as well. 'Pea' derives from the Dutch word 'pij', a type of cloth for the early version of the coat. The pea coat looks good on men of all ages. If you are of medium height, avoid long styles as they will make you look shorter. This classic coat has the ability to

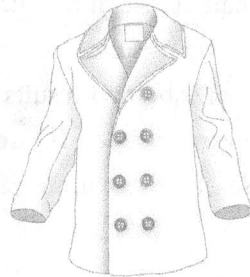

dress up a T-shirt and jeans or a checked shirt and chinos. Due to its length, I don't recommend wearing it with a suit.

In the end, the pea coat is a classic for a reason — practical function combined with great aesthetics. The simple, classic cut can be anything from casual to slightly dressy, keeping a man warm in all kinds of conditions. Its wool material wears well, holds up to abuse, and is one of the least intricate, but stylish coats ever made. Most importantly, it makes a man look good. The broad shoulders, thin waist, wide collar and double-breasted front make a man look slightly bigger, stronger, and taller than he really is — a big plus. To this day when weather permits, I still wear my navy pea coat which was purchased over 20 years ago.

Chesterfield coat

A formal coat is a 'chesterfield' named after the Sixth Earl of Chesterfield. It has no horizontal seam or sidebodies, it can be single- or double-breasted, and has been popular in a wide variety of fabrics, typically heavier weight tweeds or charcoal and navy, and even the camel hair classic. It has often been made with a velvet or fur collar. It is a formal coat that works best with suits and tuxedos, and is most definitely not your everyday coat. If purchasing a formal coat, ensure it fits over at least the two inner garments, which are your shirt and suit jacket.

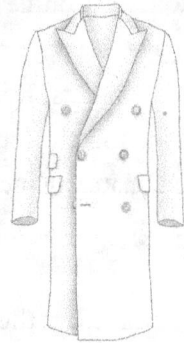

Looking after your coat

Whatever coat you decide on to keep you toasty during winter, ensure you look after it, as it will look after you:

- Hang your coat on a wooden hanger with broad-shaped shoulder pieces.
- Brush it frequently to remove foreign particles such as dust and lint.
- Have any stains removed immediately — the quicker the better — as wool stains can seep deep within.
- Give it a steam every season, either professionally, or at least hang it in the bathroom whilst taking a shower.
- Only have it dry cleaned once a year, preferably at the end of the cold season prior to storage.
- When storing long-term, place in a breathable fabric bag with a cedar ball.

Jackets

Sports jacket and blazer

The one similarity between a sports jacket and blazer is that neither garment comes with matching pants. A sports jacket is generally made of a patterned material, such as herringbone, stripes or checks and is usually made from a seasonal material like tweed, flannel, cotton or linen. Traditionally, a blazer usually means anything with pockets and comes in solid dark colours such as navy, black or grey with gold, silver or fine wool-covered buttons.

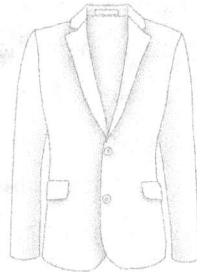

The term 'sports jacket' originated from the sport of hunting whilst experimenting with sports clothes. Men were seeking comfort and status in their clothing by the early 20th century, and turned to the ever-changing sport jacket. Its role was to add versatility to its practical side by looking the part as men chatted at the gentleman's club after a hunting event.

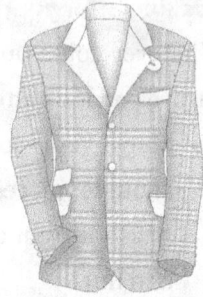

The sports jacket as we know it today has a very different role. The bold patterns and heavy fabric make it improper for business or formal occasions. It is best worn with denim jeans or chino pants and paired with a plain non-patterned shirt with both white and light blue working best.

The blazer also derives from a sporting background, in the English cricket club scene. Originally the blazer was in club colours or striped with a crest on the breast pocket. Today blazers are offered in a breadth of styles, which offer the detailed options of a flap or patch pocket, different size lapels and buttons. Keep it basic and choose the traditional navy blue blazer, as it will offer the most versatility, practicality and style within your wardrobe. Always try to complement the jacket rather than wearing something in the same colour. For example, wear denim, corduroy or chino pants with a contrasting hue such as white jeans, brown corduroy and beige-coloured chinos.

Whether wearing a sports coat or a blazer, the same principal applies — make sure it fits you properly! You want it to hug your shoulders and follow the lines of your body all the way down to your waist. A good sports jacket or blazer should make you stand up straight and feel like a winner, no matter what sport you play.

Denim trucker jacket

I was recently asked what my favourite items of clothing were and I took no time in responding with 'my denim jackets'. For as long as I can remember I have always had one, and today have accumulated over half a dozen. My range consists of different shades of colour but has always been loyal to the tried, true and tested old school brands of Lee, Wrangler, Levi and Edwin.

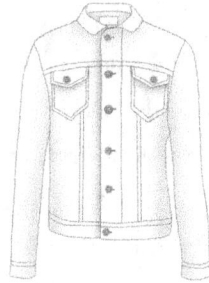

Levi introduced the riveted jacket in 1910. The real defining moment came with the introduction of the trucker jacket aimed at long haulage drivers after both Lee and Wrangler had the ranch workers market sewn up in the late 1950s. Once again Hollywood had people of influence creating supply issues with Paul Newman in Hud and Marilyn Monroe in The Misfits when both movies first aired in 1960s.

I tend to wear this icon piece most of the year. In winter I like to wear it under a sports jacket, pea coat or overcoat. It adds an unexpected, youthful edge to a traditional shirt and coat pairing. The darker and less distressed the wash, the easier it is to mix with dress shoes and tailored pants. In the warmer climates I wear it as a standalone piece matched with jeans of a different shade, chinos or cords.

Fit is important. Stay with old-school brands and keep it simple. Stay away from smoke and mirror designs, washes, buckles and buttons.

Just make sure your jacket and jeans are several shades apart, otherwise you run the risk of looking like a denim advertisement. Dark, crisp jeans, for instance, should be paired with a worn, light-coloured jacket. The shades or wash need to be significantly different to give separation. 'Double denim' as it is known when one wears denim on the top and bottom halves of the body has long been one of my favorite combinations to wear. I have done so for years despite it being frowned upon by some fashion critics. In the summertime I find it the perfect weight when the temperature cools down. Pair with any type of shorts and a plain T-shirt and deck shoes, runners or thongs, and you are ready for action.

Bing Crosby was refused entry to an upmarket hotel during the 1950s because he was wearing a denim jacket, so Levi Strauss made him a denim tuxedo. He re-entered the hotel a week later and was granted a VIP life membership. Long live the power of denim!

Rebel without a cause: The leather jacket

What did Marlon Brando, Steve McQueen, John Travolta and Fonzie all have in common? They were the cool dudes who made leather jackets iconic. They took the punk and bikie stigma of the leather jacket to a new 'cool' with their respective roles in On the Waterfront, The Great Escape, Grease and Happy Days.

Before these guys, the tough image of the leather jacket started with the leather bomber jackets created for the US Air Force. The leather kept pilots warm during a time when cockpits were not enclosed. The original leather jackets were constructed to act as a second skin and protect the body not only from the elements, but also from major cuts and bruises, which were a part of going to war.

Due to its excellent resistance to abrasion and wind, as soon as motorcycles were invented most riders took to wearing heavy leather jackets to protect themselves from injury. Top-quality motorcycle leather is superior to any man-made fabric for abrasion protection, which is why it is still used in racing today.

There are two points I would like to make clear about a leather jacket. Firstly they are one of the few investment pieces you should buy, and secondly they are the one thing you should never, ever throw out. It's a fantastic item to anchor other trend pieces that will be in for a season and then out the next.

If you're in the market to buy a new leather jacket, spend extra for high quality leather. For versatility and timeless trends, stick to the traditional black or brown leather. Ensure it is fitted and make sure it ends no higher than the top of your pants, without excess material around the stomach and chest.

It should hug your shoulders, not slouch off them. Avoid all the bells and whistles; this includes distressed leather, padded elbows and racing stripes.

As leather is a natural fibre it needs to breathe, so store it in a cool, dry space when you're not wearing it. Purchase a leather protector spray; it will help if any unwanted stains occur.

All fashion is cyclical and if you were one of those guys that purchased the 1980s George Michael short leather jacket complete with encrusted silver studs, then hang tough, your day might yet arrive again. When it does, I will let you know!

If the shoe fits ...

As the old saying goes, "You can tell the measure of a man by his shoes".

Shoes are often the most overlooked item in a man's wardrobe, yet arguably the most important. They say a lot about your personality and attention to detail, and can be the difference between looking average or looking immaculate.

Durability, comfort, style and sophistication are what you get when purchasing a high-grade pair of shoes. Good quality workmanship, material, detail and design will come at a price but is an investment when compared to the mass-produced cheaper counterparts, which will need to be replaced on a regular basis.

Luxurious shoes are usually handmade, a timely process that can have more than a dozen people tanning, cutting and stitching to guarantee a flawless finish. This process will ensure less machine manufacturing mistakes, coupled with a more detailed long-lasting finish.

Buying quality leather-crafted shoes will definitely help enhance a man's image, as lower priced imitations are associated with a lack of style, taste and imagination — things which women find most unattractive. Women will evaluate and make judgements about a man by viewing his shoes as they are the 'handbag' of the ensemble in their eyes.

Due to the contrast it creates, poor quality shoes are very noticeable when a man is well dressed. Therefore it is far better to have four pairs of quality shoes than ten pairs of average shoes. No matter what else you are wearing, how good it looks and how much it all costs, poor quality shoes will have the last say and what will be remembered. There is no substitute for real leather and suede, no matter how shiny the vinyl or plastic whilst in the shoe shop.

To build the perfect stylish wardrobe for any occasion the five types of shoes to invest in are: loafers, brogues, monk straps, wing-tip oxfords and boat shoes.

Loafers

The loafer is a slip on shoe which has no laces, buckles or fastening features. Manufactured from leather or suede, they resemble a moccasin-shaped top and a flat heel. Some loafers will have a tassel or strap on the top for decoration. Every bit as sharp as a dress shoe but easy to slip on, loafers can be found in a variety of styles. Versatility is the key by offering the perfect compromise between dressy and casual. Team them with chinos, dark jeans, tailored shorts, dress pants and a slim-fit suit.

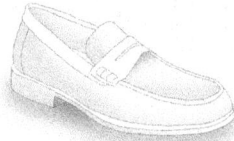

Brogues

Brogues are recognised by their decorative perforated leather and lace-up fastening, and can be worn as an alternative to the dress shoe. Their renewed popularity means they are available in a variety of colours and finishes, as well as the two-tone spectator style commonly worn by gangsters in the Prohibition era. Team with dress pants, dark denim, tailored shorts, a suit or even a tuxedo.

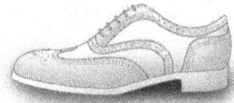

Monk straps

Monk Straps are a more dressed-up loafer, and are distinguishable by a single or double buckle-and-strap closure on the outside of the shoe. They are elegant and well designed, but not suitable for formal occasions or business despite the leather or suede finish. Team these with a casual suit, dress pants, dark jeans and chinos.

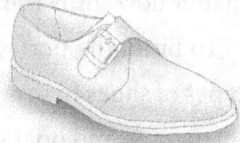

Oxfords

Oxfords are a simply-designed low-cut shoe which lace up the front. They have flat heels and thin soles. Some oxfords have a separate piece of leather on the toe known as a 'cap toe'. The 'wingtip' is arguably the most common of all oxfords. This is recognisable by toe 'brogue-ing' that resembles a bird with its wings spread. Team these with double-breasted and pinstripe suits, tweed jackets, dress trousers, chinos and dark jeans.

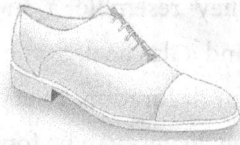

Boat shoes

Boat shoes, deck shoes or top-siders, as they are also known, are leather or canvas shoes with rubber soles. They are manufactured by hundreds of different companies offering a huge range in colours and slight variations on design. Versatility is the shoe's strength, as they can be worn with short or long pants. Team with all type of shorts, linen pants, chinos, jeans and cargo pants.

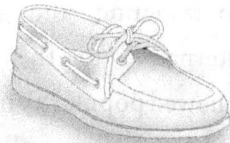

Caring for your shoes

When owning shoes such as those listed above, proper care is not just about appearance, it's also about preserving and adding life while protecting your investment. Without sufficient care, leather can dry out until it eventually cracks, leaving the shoe unwearable.

- Always use a shoehorn when putting on your shoes. This will keep the backs strong and sturdy.
- Try to wear your shoes in dry conditions for the first few occasions.
- Fine leather shoes can require a full day to dry out from natural perspiration. Try to give them at least 24 hours between wears.
- Try to avoid excessive wetting. Should this occur, always let the shoes dry naturally away from direct heat. Use newspaper inside the shoe to help the leather dry out.
- Your shoes will benefit from regular use of a good quality cream or wax polish. This helps to moisturise the leather, as well as to prevent cracking and excessive creasing.

To maintain your shoes in great condition, the four steps are: clean, condition, polish and waterproof.

- Start by removing any excess dirt with a gentle leather cleaner or saddle soap using a brush to eliminate dirt in those hard to get places.
- Rub on a small amount of leather conditioner until the shoe has an even applied coat. Wipe off any excess after a few minutes, as the shoe will only absorb what it needs.
- Apply the correct colour shoe polish and buff off with a soft cloth or a pantyhose.
- Waterproof your shoes with a specific waterproofing agent,

but wipe the shoes lightly with a warm sponge beforehand to make the shoe more porous and improve its ability to absorb the product.

You will be judged by your shoes, so take the time to find a quality pair that suits your style and lifestyle, and then look after them — they are worth every cent and bit of care.

Run Forrest, run: The sneaker

Sneakers or sandshoes of yesteryear were only required as part of a man's exercise attire, and the more colourful and flashy they were, the faster they went (or so I thought). In today's fast-paced times we need to invest in at least two pairs of sneakers — the exercise pair and the versatile casual pair.

Exercise shoes should provide support and comfort, which is best achieved by correct fitting from an expert. Sports shops today offer a service to ensure the correct sneakers are chosen for your height, weight, and most importantly, your gait. If your feet turn inwards or outwards, the correct support and comfort in the shoe will be essential.

A correctly-fitted athletic shoe is a necessity to your physical wellbeing and comfort, and you will kick yourself if you don't do it. You will discover some exercise shoes look better suited to a futuristic space mission than a jog in the park, but some of those colourful-looking hip features can also serve a purpose.

Exercise shoes are probably the most important piece of fitness equipment you'll buy, so it's imperative to choose the right pair. Ensure your sales assistant is knowledgeable and they go through the correct procedure to get the correct shoe for your weight, gait and amount of activity intended. Speciality running shops offer a great service by viewing your running style and landing pattern, then subsequently selecting the perfect shoe. This is well worth it.

The casual pair needs to be comfortable, versatile and look good. Here are some tips to ensure all three bases are covered:

- Hightops have slowly made their way onto the streets again, but if you are over the age of 16 do not even attempt to wear these.

- Choose the basic, low-cut lace-up without any offensive colours and glitz — these elements can be added through accessories such as scarves, a coloured polo or striped tie — best to keep the wheels simple. One basic colour goes with everything from jeans and chinos to shorts. You can dress up the look with a blazer, or keep it classic coupled with a polo shirt. Colours such as navy, neutral shades and white offer the best value.

- Invisible ankle socks or very low-cut socks are the best option. Once you have unnoticeable socks, feel free to go for a pair of chinos or jeans with the cuffs rolled up. This look can be an alternative to a leather dress shoe on a casual Friday at the office. It's the perfect way to kick off the weekend a little earlier and go straight to after-work drinks.

- Steer clear of over-designed casual shoes — keep them basic and simple. As with sneakers keep the footwear simple, if you want to add need colour to your outfit then do so with a scarf, pastel polo shirt or striped tie.

Sock it to 'em

You may only think of socks at Christmas when the mother-in-law very thoughtfully passes over the beautifully wrapped standard three-pack as your regular gift. This small and what we think of as an 'unseen' necessity could be the culprit that spoils a perfectly considered dapper outfit.

To make sure your outfit does not fall into this category, cast your eye over these basics:

Socks fall into three categories: dress, casual and sports. The most common mistake is wearing sport socks (often white) with casual and dress outfits. We can often forget that each time we sit down, at least eight centimetres of sock will be seen. White socks are best left for outdoor sporting activities and should not be pulled up to maximum length.

When wearing dress or casual pants, the colour of your socks should be dictated by the colour of your pants and not by the shade of your shoes. Black pants should go with black socks, and brown pants with brown socks.

The reason it is important to match socks with pants is the sock exposure when sitting down. Co-ordination will give a more fluid appearance.

Once you have the basic sock-matching, you can incorporate subtle patterns and colours. By this I mean if you are wearing a black suit with black shoes and a red tie, try black socks with a red pattern. Remember subtlety is the key.

When wearing jeans, stay with dark-coloured socks such as navy and charcoal. And for the record, novelty socks, socks in bed and socks with sandals are just not on — no exceptions!

Reg Grundies: The importance of underwear

I was blown away not long ago when reading an article that stated men take eight years to replace their underwear. Guys, that is one bad habit and a real crook look. Once your 'Reg Grundies' have a hole, lose their elasticity, become frayed, are stained or no longer fit, it is time to move on! Just because you think no one will see them or Grandma will gift wrap a pack of six in primary colours for her usual birthday gift, take ownership now and don't become a statistic.

You should have at least ten pairs of undies on hand at all times. That's one for every day of the week plus two additional pairs for weekend nights and another thrown in for good measure. Find a brand that's comfortable and makes you feel confident, and then stock up.

It's also important to have an assortment of underwear for various activities. Briefs provide the right support for almost every situation from work to play, but sometimes you just need to set things free come bedtime with a looser-fitting boxer. Whatever you wear, just ensure they are worn no longer than 12 hours and are washed after every wear.

Call it what you want, 'living large' or 'hanging loose,' but opting out of undies is never acceptable unless you are sleeping. We all know what the consequences would be of not having that extra layer of material between 'that area' and the metal fly. There is an abundance of underwear styles, makes, cuts, colours and brands so please just ensure you purchase on a regular basis and keep them concealed. Showing your undies logo band was semi-cool in the early '90s, but they are best tucked away. Live by the motto, 'the better your underwear looks on, the greater the chance someone will want to take them off'.

Chapter 3:
Accessorise

Dead heat: The tie and how to tie it

It is amazing the amount of power a piece of material five centimetres wide and 50 centimetres long can have, and what that material says about your personality, profession and personal style. I am talking about the tie, or 'dead heat' as I sometimes refer to it. Just wearing a tie does not automatically enhance your status, but choosing the right tie can be an important step on your road to riches, whether work- or personally-related.

The staple white or pale blue business shirt offers the most versatility when matching with a tie. Solid coloured ties like navy, charcoal, burgundy and black are the safest bet when pairing with blue, grey and black suits. Solids are striking, elegant and classy when they are made of good material, of which, pure silk is by far the best.

Do not be afraid to pair your tie and shirt in different shades of the same colour, such as navy and pale blue or charcoal and grey, as the subtle contrast gives a contemporary and elegant look.

When in a business environment and needing an edge in a presentation, a solid crimson tie has the biggest impact in people's memories.

When incorporating stripes into the mix, as a general rule, you can wear a striped shirt with a striped tie, but ensure the stripes aren't identical in size. When wearing this combination, make sure at least one colour in your tie matches either your suit and/or shirt. Avoid wearing a striped shirt with a striped tie and a pinstriped suit as you will resemble the 100 metres athletic track with so many lines!

The same principles apply for a check pattern, make sure there is a contrast in check size and one colour in the tie matches with the shirt or suit.

The safest bet in regards to width for a tie is around 7.5 centimetres, and anything in this vicinity will always be in style. Trends for skinny ties and wide ties will come and go, but it's best to experiment with colours and patterns and leave the sizing to the sports stars, rappers and rock stars.

A good trait for a quality tie is one that has been cut across the fabric. This will allow the tie to fall straight down after the knot has been tied. It's best to stay away from flashing lights, cartoon characters and sports emblems if you need to be taken seriously or if you're attending a wedding or funeral.

Tie Knots

Here are four classic knots suitable for business, personal and special occasions:

Double Windsor

This is a wide triangular knot usually worn for formal occasions, but being all-purpose it is also appropriate for meetings and interviews. This type of knot looks best worn with a shirt collar considerably cut-away.

Here is how it is made:

1. Drape the necktie around your collar and start with the wider end extending approximately 30 centimetres below the arrow end, then cross it over.

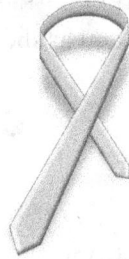

2. Wrap the wide end around and bring it up and over, then through the loop between the collar and the tie. Pull it down towards the front.

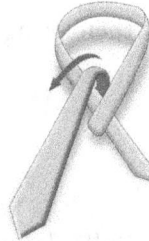

3. Curl what is left of the wide end behind the narrow end.

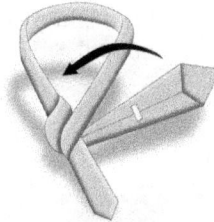

4. Bring the wide end back up again through the loop.

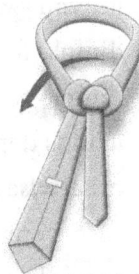

5. Put down through the loop and pull around across the narrow end as shown.

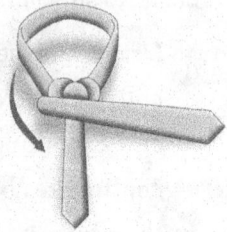

6. Bring the wide end up and tuck it through the loop a third time, then bring it back down to the front.

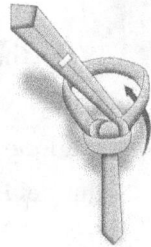

7. Pull down on the wide end carefully to tighten. Draw up the knot snugly to your collar.

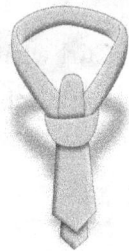

8. Finish your knot by tightening it; you will see the start of a dimple forming. Manipulate the dimple to make it noticeable, as it adds depth and character to an otherwise drab flat surface. Make sure your collar falls nicely all around, and centre the knot as best you can.

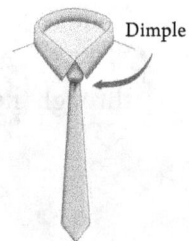

Dimple

Four-In-Hand

This quick, easy and highly popular knot can be worn for all occasions but is best suited to a more casual look. It works best with wide ties made from heavy fabrics and should be worn with a tab, button-down or regular spread collar.

1. Drape the necktie around your collar and start with the wider end extending approximately 30 centimetres below the narrow end. Cross it over.

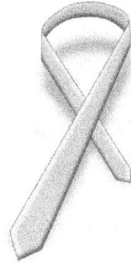

2. Wrap the wide end underneath the narrow end. Continue by bringing the wide end back over in front of the narrow end again.

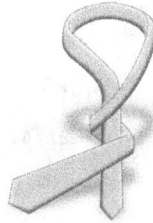

3. Pull the wide end up and through the back of the loop. Hold the front of the knot loose with your index finger and pass the wide end down through the loop.

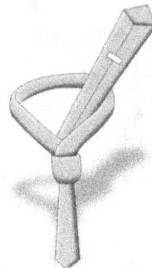

4. Complete the knot by tightening
    it.

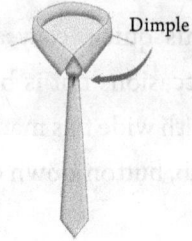

Dimple

Half-Windsor

The little brother of the Windsor, the Half-Windsor is a medium triangular knot suitable for more formal settings than the Four-In-Hand. It can be worn for any occasion, is compatible with standard shirt collars, and works best with somewhat wider ties made from light to medium fabrics.

1. Drape the necktie around your collar and start with the wider end extending approximately 30 centimetres below the narrow one. Cross the wider section over the narrow end to form an X-shape.

2. Bring the wide end up through the loop and then back down.

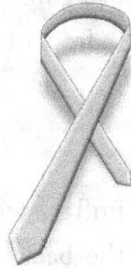

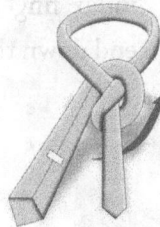

3.   Wrap the wide end back around
     to the front.

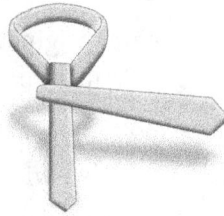

4.   Swing it back up through the loop
     again.

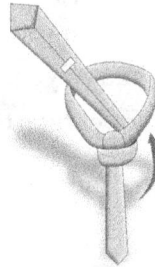

5.   Carefully pull the wide end all the
     way through and tighten the knot.

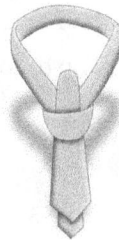

6.   Hold the narrow end, push up the
     knot, and tighten it snugly around
     your collar. Manipulate to get the
     dimple.

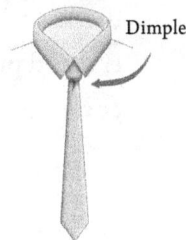

Dimple

Pratt (Shelby) Knot

This knot was originated in the late '80s by Jerry Pratt, who worked for the US Chamber of Commerce, but it was made infamous by Minneapolis news anchor Don Shelby. A 92-year-old viewer who was disgruntled with Shelby's atrocious on-air tie knots showed him how to tie the new knot.

1. Start with the tie inside out, front side toward your neck and wide end on your right, 30 centimetres lower than the narrow end.

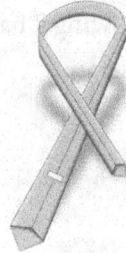

2. Take the wide end over and under the narrow end and through the loop to form a knot.

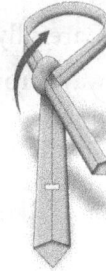

3. Pull both ends apart to ensure the knot is tight. Take the wide end and pull it across to the right, covering your first knot.

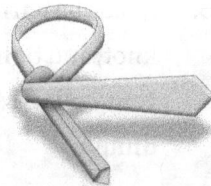

4. Pull the wide end under the loop of the knot.

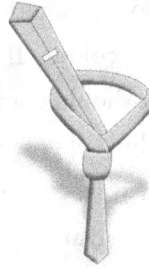

5. Drop the wide end through the loop to form the knot. Tighten, creating the dimple.

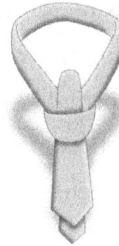

Think outside the square:
The pocket square & how to fold it

A simple, stylish and inexpensive way to go from drab to dapper is a piece of fabric in the top jacket pocket — better known as the 'pocket square'. When added to an outfit, this small accessory allows men to express themselves and vary their look without having to spend too much.

It is said the pocket square originated with English and French noblemen. They carried perfumed and embroidered hankies in order to cover their noses from the stench of the streets and other people. Thankfully, we 21st century men smell like roses so they only serve an aesthetic purpose these days. Do not use it to wipe or blow your nose!

A pocket square is best made of silk and can be patterned or solid in colour. The general guideline is that your pocket square colour should complement some colour on your tie, so if your tie has a hint of green, choose a pocket square in solid green. Never match your tie colour or pattern completely, as it will look too structured and obvious — like you are trying too hard.

You do not need to wear a tie to wear a pocket square; in fact a pocket square can be a good substitute for a tie. It adds enough detail and individual creativity for any occasion that is not black tie or formal. A pocket square can be worn a number of ways, which all comes down to personal taste. Here are five square-folding techniques to see you on your way:

The Four Point

1. Lay your pocket square flat with one corner facing up and one corner facing down, so it is a diamond shape.

2. Fold the bottom corner up to meet the top corner.

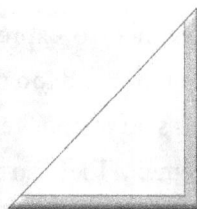

3. Fold the bottom corner up to the top, just to the left of the top corner.

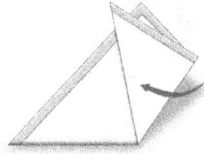

4. Fold the left side towards the right, and up to the right of the middle point of the crown.

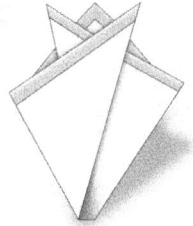

5. Turn the pocket square around and adjust the points of the crown. Place in your jacket pocket.

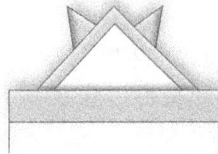

The One Point/Triangle

1. Lay the pocket square flat.

2. Fold it in half lengthwise.

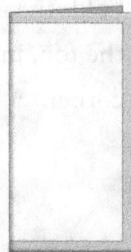

3. Fold it again from bottom to top
    to form the perfect square.

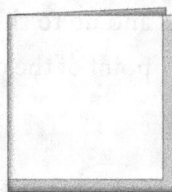

4. Move the square to make a
    diamond shape. Fold the left
    corner to the middle of the
    diamond.

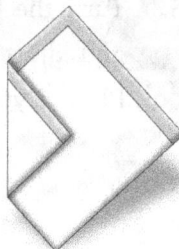

5. Fold the right corner to overlap
    the left fold just a little. Fold the
    bottom corner back to show the
    last two folds.

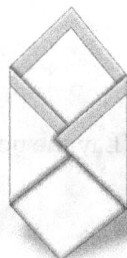

6.   Tuck into pocket, exposing 3–4 centimetres.

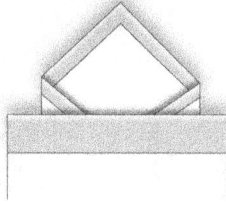

The Square/Presidential

1.   Lay your pocket square flat.

2.   Fold the left side over the right side.

3.   Fold the bottom up, just short of the top.

4. Flip it around and tuck as needed, and place in your jacket pocket.

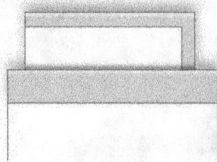

The Puff

1. Lay the pocket square flat.

2. Pinch the middle of the pocket square and pick it up, letting it hang naturally.

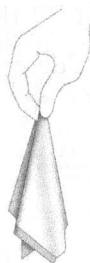

3. Forming a circle with your thumb and forefinger, clasp the hanging square at the midway point.

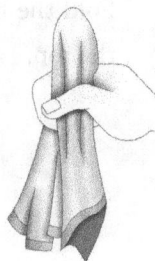

4. Fold up the excess material below the hand, and stuff inside the jacket pocket, revealing 2–3 centimetres.

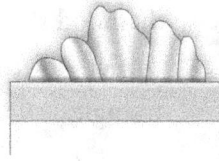

The TV Fold

1. Lay the pocket square flat.

2. Fold it in half lengthwise.

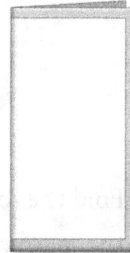

3. Fold it again from bottom to top to form the perfect square.

4. Move the square to form a diamond shape. Fold the bottom corner to the top to form a triangle.

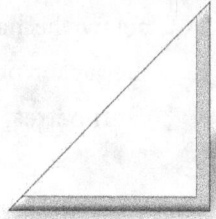

5. Fold the left corner over just past the middle.

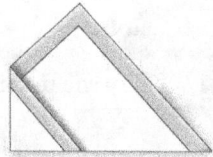

6. Fold the right corner over to overlap.

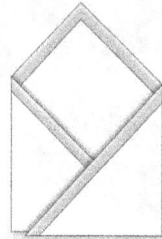

7. Fold the top corner down to form the perfect square. Flip it over to hide the diagonal folds. Place in jacket pocket to reveal 1–2 centimetres.

Belt up tight: The right belt

The belt is the most overlooked accessory, but an absolute necessity in a man's wardrobe. Don't spend big bucks on your professional and casual wardrobe, but then neglect the importance of what a belt can say and do.

Every man should own five belts: a black and a brown, a formal dress belt and two casual belts. Formal dress belts are around the width of your thumb and have a glossy finish. The casual belt is wider, typically in a matte finish and in varying textures, styles and materials.

The simplest rule to follow when wearing a formal dress belt is that it should be the same colour as your shoes. Casual belts allow more flexibility, which is why I suggest having two. A brown or tan belt around four centimetres wide will offer the most versatility. Whether paired with sneakers, boots or casual shoes, a tan colour will cover all options in the casual wear stakes.

For a more colourful and individual look, a striped canvas belt is the perfect touch. It provides a great way to break up an outfit in a cool way without being too noticeable.

Top 5 Belt Tips

Here are 5 simple things you need to remember about belts:

- Leave the bling, beads and big fancy buckles to the girls and cowboys at the rodeo.
- Never wear a formal dress belt with jeans, or a casual belt with formal pants.
- Ensure your belts are of good leather, or you will have to replace them regularly. Groove marks become prominent and are highly noticeable when you need to use another hole.

While on holes, never punch your own. It's like cutting your own hair — highly obvious.

- When buying a belt, measure your waist and go one size bigger. Don't make the mistake of not wearing a belt; you are not fully dressed without one.
- Only wear a belt with shorts when golfing, sailing or at the retirement village.

Layer upon layer: Layering your clothing

When the cooler weather is upon us it means grey skies, cold winds, runny red noses and storing those beloved boardies for the next three months. The positives? Rain on the roof when you are lying in bed, a roaring fire and layering clothes.

Layering is dressing in numerous garments, which are worn over each other for practical or aesthetic reasons. There are no rules when it comes to layering, but a cold climate lends itself to three layers when it comes to showcasing your personal style and regulating body temperature.

Your first layer should act like a second skin: a cotton singlet or white T-shirt. Second layers, such as a shirt, provide additional insulation, leaving a little of the first layer to peek through.

A third layer protects you from the elements and pulls your whole look together. This is the most important layer since it is the most visible. The easiest way to layer is with a blazer jacket, but there are many other options as well, such as vests, cardigans or V-neck sweaters.

An important rule to remember is to avoid large, bulky, oversized garments altogether. The purpose of layering is to create a warm, sophisticated look that is both smooth and complementary. Layering pieces that are too big or too bulky will only defeat the purpose.

When layering your look, start with lightweight fabrics underneath and heavier ones on top. When wearing layers, you should build gradually in terms of weight from the inside out. This will help with warmth, comfort and the finished look. Always be wary of layering multiple patterns like stripes and checks together. Wear complementary colours to balance the overall appearance of their final look. Using this method ensures all the layers in the outfit work together. The best layering tip for casual clothes in winter is to use a hoodie as a second layer, as it looks cool under a jacket and the hood comes in handy for warmth and wind protection.

Accessories such as hats and scarves can add colour and vibrancy to a winter's day, but ensure they are plain if your outer layer is busy and patterned. Don't be afraid to wear a scarf — just make sure it is applied the correct way which I discuss in the next chapter.

Scarf theory & knots: Scarves & how to tie them

Not only do scarves serve the obvious purpose of keeping you warm, they are the perfect accessory to add life and individuality to your outfit.

When matching a scarf to your outfit, ensure even the slightest hint of colour can be found elsewhere within your outfit. Also remember only one bold piece per outfit, so go easy on the pattern, texture and colours if your jacket, shirt or hat is playing the striking centrepiece.

Stay with natural fibres like merino wool, alpaca, pashmina and cashmere for winter warmth. For warmer climates stay with silk, cotton and linen.

How to Wear a Scarf

Here are the four manliest ways to wear a scarf:

The Parisian

Place the scarf in both hands and fold it over lengthwise. Drape it around your neck, insert the loose ends through the loop hanging in front of you. Pull the ends through.

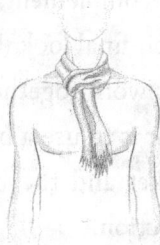

The Once-A

Place the scarf around your neck allowing one end of the scarf to be longer than the other. Take the long end and bring it around your neck and let it fall over your chest.

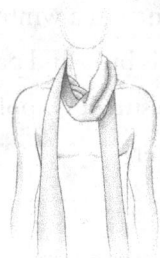

The Loosey

The same rules apply as above — just let it hang loosely like you have been a little short of time to finish it off. This is a casual version of the Once–A.

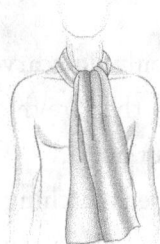

The Twice-A

Start as you would with the Once-A, but make sure one end of the scarf is significantly longer than the other. Take the much longer end and circle it around your neck twice; do this without making the knot look like you are being strangled.

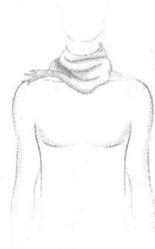

You can leave your hat on: Choosing a hat

I must confess my interest in hats has increased recently, not only because of the climatic benefits and environmental precautions, but more so since my own 'hair hat' dwindled, receded and slowly vanished.

Hats are the perfect way to mix up a look while providing all the warmth or shade required. The fashion of wearing hats, popular during the '30s to '60s when men were sharply dressed, is slowly making its way back in vogue, so I thought it best to pass on some hat advice for you lucky men with long, thick locks — and for those without.

My top five picks are as follows:

- A flat cap and newsboy hat can be associated with older men, but when worn with casual clothing such as a denim jacket, varsity jacket, hoodie or windcheater it offers a great style and look. A Harris Tweed pattern or a grey check will offer the most variety when pairing with casual clothes.

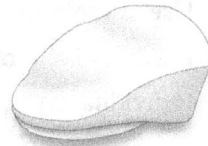

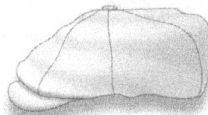

- When the occasion to dress up arrives, the walking hat is all class and style. It is the larger cousin of the fedora hat and came to prominence in the iconic film *The Godfather*. It is best paired with a suit, tie and trench coat, with black the best colour.

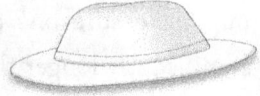

- A beanie is a must-have item, and the jack-of-all-trades in the cooler weather. Both fitted and slouchy beanies can be worn with any outfit, offering individual style through colour and pattern. My only advice is no pom-poms or footy logos.

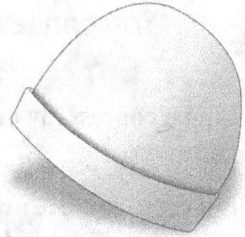

- A good straw Panama hat is a must for the summer months, offering style, comfort, protection and an all-round classy look. This hat can be worn with suits, casual clothing at a barbecue, shorts and at the beach. Use a coloured-band around the outside of the hat to suit your own individual style.

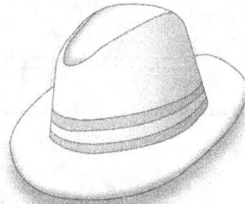

- A cap is a necessity for outdoor house chores and when exercising. There is a plethora of caps available in various materials, colours, logos, styles and shapes. Wear one that is comfortable and not too outlandish. When branded, ensure it is a brand you like to be associated with and keep the logo to a minimum. Do not attempt to wear it like a rap star.

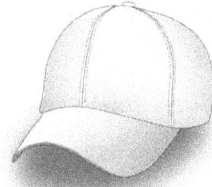

Hat Etiquette

Always remember that the correct hat etiquette is to remove it whenever you're inside, partaking in the national anthem, being photographed and at all introductions. Once removed, hold your hat in such a way that only the outside (never the lining) is visible.

It's in the bag, man: Choosing the classic bag

What once was considered only a female accessory has now become a necessary style accessory for men. This is mainly due to the ever-increasing list of items and gadgets required when leaving the house. The bag is back and it has come a long way since the infamous 'man bag' of the '80s.

Here are six stylish options for business and casual to help ease the burden, and for that matter, the very bad look of full pockets.

Briefcase

The briefcase is probably the most traditional and 'acceptable' form of bag for men. Modern briefcases have evolved a great deal since the days of your grandfather's with the secret combination lock. The use of high quality leather and colours make this a great option for those who work in an office.

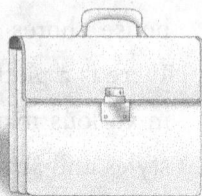

Messenger

The messenger bag made from canvas or leather and swung across the shoulder has taken on a whole new meaning in male fashion. Its laidback style will always have a classic, casual look with a hint of business sophistication.

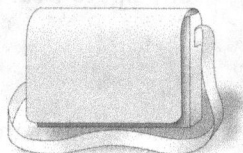

Holdall

The holdall is for those weekend getaways or three-day trips. No more cumbersome, heavy sports bags, its design is inspired by the duffel bag, but its mostly leather exterior and more refined appearance contribute to a classic look. It is a practical all-rounder.

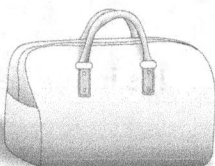

Camera Bag

The camera bag is a smaller version of the messenger bag; good for any man on the go. It is a discreet but severely stylish way to lug around your belongings.

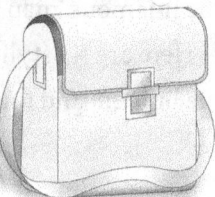

Tote

The tote is the hip approach to the classic briefcase, and is the pinnacle in casual business attire. Its basic design and usually soft leather exterior allows it a classic status, while its long handles give it a contemporary edge.

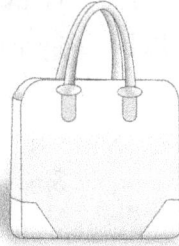

Newsboy

The newsboy bag is a classic style synonymous with men's casual wear. It's similar to the messenger bag but less formal, as it is made from canvas material. This bag style is perfect for everyday use and is the backpack of today.

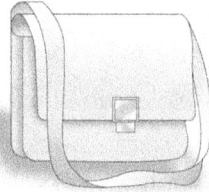

For a number of years now I have had a brown leather messenger bag. Inside you will find the communication necessities required today, plus a pad and pen, a packet of chewies, a handkerchief and two band aids for those unexpected little emergencies.

Invest your money wisely: Buying a wallet

I must confess I was always more concerned with what was inside my wallet than how it appeared from the outside, until what I thought would be a quick 'in and out' shopping experience to purchase a new one. I suddenly realised that size, material, colour, compartments and logos are all important when searching for this often overlooked necessity. A good wallet not only has plenty in it, but should make it easy for its owner to locate their money and cards, be easily accessible and properly organised.

Wallets are not a reflection of your fashion sense, but with a little research and time it is possible to be practical as well as fashionable. Since your wallet will on average last three years, why not purchase a quality, stylish one?

Whether sporty or more traditional, wallets are available in fashionable styles and colours with enough variety to suit everyone's taste.

The more casual sporty wallet is usually made from lightweight nylon, twill, vinyl or rubber in an assortment of colours, shapes and sizes. The closure mechanism is generally Velcro or a zip. Surf brands made this type of wallet their own due to the waterproof material and the casual look. High-end designer brands have also jumped on the trend with this type of style, but my advice is to keep the flashy logo to a minimum.

The more traditional wallet is generally made of leather, which comes in varying shapes and sizes. The most traditional and timeless option is the bi-fold wallet, which consists of eight card slots plus two flat pockets, which should be sufficient to carry all of your important cards and hard earned cash. This style can also be purchased as a tri-fold if you need more space.

Empty your wallet weekly of all unnecessary receipts and stubs; a thick wallet in the back pocket is no longer a sign of excess cash. I tried this for years when $1 and $2 notes were around — a $20 and a $50 either side of the big bunch worked in the '80s, or so I thought. Now I find my loose change is a goldmine for the kids.

The sporty-type wallet is best for active men, brown leather for the outdoorsy type, and black leather for the corporate type. Stay away from too much bling and logos; pay extra for quality leather and work hard to keep it full of the folding stuff.

Time is ticking: Choosing a watch

For those who have a gift certificate, some leftover cash (half your luck) or just want to spoil themselves when the Christmas presents they got were not up to scratch, a good item to invest in is a watch.

With everyone carrying a mobile phone, why buy a watch? Because it is an investment, a statement, and is the only piece of jewellery a man needs to wear.

A man's watch can give us a peek into his character, style, taste, personality and background, so it's best you take the time (no pun intended) in choosing the right one. Only a select few can be in the market for a premium watch, but we can all have a better understanding of them.

An analogue watch has a face that holds hour and minute hands, and either numbers, markers or Roman numerals that display a 12-hour day. It is considered formal.

Another element that separates watches is how they are powered. Digital watches are powered by an ultra-small battery. With either an LCD or LED face that displays the time in numeric form. Digital watches are better teamed with casual clothes. Quartz watches are analogue devices that run on a tiny, vibrating, electrified quartz crystal. Mechanical watches are powered by a complex array of finely tuned parts. These watches are at the high end of the price range due to the craftsmanship involved.

In relation to colour, silver watches match best with blacks, greys, silvers and blues. Ideally you should wear them at night.

Gold watches go with browns, beiges, tans and other earth tones. These are best worn during the day.

No matter the type, style or colour, your watch should fit firmly without leaving an imprint on your wrist.

I bought my Seiko diving watch with a black plastic band for my 21st birthday in Tokyo a quarter of a century ago and it still works, so quality will withstand the test of time.

Watch Tips

Here are my top tips for wearing a watch:

- A watch should be worn securely. It is not a bracelet.
- There is a difference between waterproof and water-resistant, don't learn the hard way.
- Don't expose your watch to the extremes of hot and cold climatic conditions.
- Air out leather strap watches every few day or run the risk of smelling like a wet dog.
- Similar to your car, watches works best when serviced. I would recommend at least every few years.

Raise your glasses: The right glasses for you

Regardless of your age or where you live, sunglasses are a required part of every man's life. Protection is the main purpose, but this accessory is also a fashion staple.

Choosing the right shape for your face and frame colour for your complexion could be the difference between looking like Brad Pitt or Dame Edna. These simple tips for both spectacles and sunglasses will lead you in the right direction:

- A round face is better suited to darker coloured frames. Stay with straight-angle rectangular or square frames. Thin metal frames are an option.

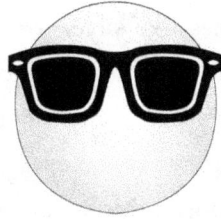

- A square face will balance better with rounded frames to level out your face. Stay clear of rectangular frames, as they will accentuate the squareness of your face shape.

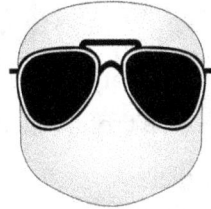

- For a triangular face you need to downplay the width at the top of your face, so thin-rimmed frames are best.

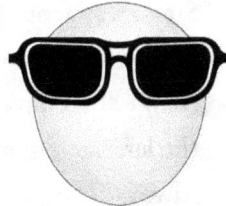

- An oval face has more options, but stay away from narrow frames as they can make your face look longer.

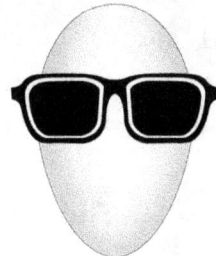

To complement hair colour, blonds are better suited to earthy toned frames. Men with dark hair have a wide scope and can explore warmer tones like bronze and gold for winter and cooler tones like silver for summer. Redheads should avoid silver and gold colours and choose warmer earthy tones like tortoiseshell. Grey-haired men should aim for pewter and metal.

They say the eyes are windows to the soul, so take the time to choose correctly and ensure they fit well. Remember, they are the first thing people see.

Glasses Tips

Here is what you need to know about wearing glasses:

- Don't rotate them upwards so they're sitting on top of on your head.
- Never wear them indoors or at night, unless you have won a Grammy award.
- Stay away from pink or yellow-tinted lenses unless you are going to a fancy dress party.
- If you don't have a case, place them in your top pocket with the lens facing inwards for protection.
- Always take your glasses off when speaking to anyone who isn't wearing any (it's a trust thing).

My goggles of choice for years have been Ray-Ban aviators for everyday use and tortoiseshell Persol for those special occasions.

The family jewels: Men's jewellery

I find it amusing and very entertaining when watching music videos to see the 155 kilos of gold jewellery draped around a rap singer and his posse. In the world of entertainment where image and branding are sometimes more important than the created sound, this look is engineered to promote the perception of wealth and success.

Observing people while out for a bite to eat and a movie recently, I was amazed to see so many men emulating RUN–D.M.C, 50 Cent and Lil Wayne without the MTV cameras present. The gold industrial-sized chains around necks and wrists, coupled with rings the size of boulders was extraordinary.

There is no bigger rap fan than myself; my newly acquired beat cube plays rap all day to the delight of my kids and the frustration of my wife. But guys, the time has arrived where the often over-used saying must now take effect — less is more. When it comes to men and jewellery, minimalism is the key.

Apart from the necessity of a watch to tell the time and add individuality to your style, here are my suggestions:

- Rings: An elegant band with no bells and whistles in the way of stones or engravings, and one ring per ten fingers.
- Bracelets: A chain around your wrist is just passable if it is slimline, elegant and doesn't clash with your watch. Beads and leather are OK when worn in a casual environment but not with formal wear or business attire.
- Necklaces: Simplicity is the key. A slimline chain with a pendant can be worn on the inside of clothing at all times. Beads and leather are also OK if worn on the inside of clothing, and when wearing shirts the two-button rule applies (that is, only leave the first top two buttons undone).
- Earrings and piercings: Leave it for the girls. Under no circumstances should men have piercings unless they are under 20-years-old, singing at night and surfing during the day. Any man of any age not living that life, take them out

now. It's OK (advisable, even) to change your style as your life experience grows.

I wear a watch and a leather-and-bead bracelet occasionally. Remember, however, that what looks good through your eyes may not seem so through others'. Ostentatious gold jewellery is not a sign of wealth — it is getting you attention for all the wrong reasons.

Chapter 4:
Dress and Act for the Occasion

Da dress code: Dress code etiquette

The most common question clients ask me about is dress code. When that invitation arrives it can be daunting trying to decode the dress code. Black tie, formal, cocktail, lounge suit, smart-casual: what does it mean and what should I wear? Overdressing can make you feel out of place, while being under-dressed can appear rude and thoughtless, and leave you feeling a little inferior.

If you're attending a formal event or your invitation reads 'black tie' it means you're required to wear a tuxedo. Today's fashion is more flexible than yesteryear. A black single-breasted model will be appropriate for most black tie events. If you want to appear more conservative, choose a double-breasted number. Your pants should never be cuffed and should always have a black satin stripe or braid running down the outside seam. A white shirt with a turn-down collar coupled with a black bow tie is the most classic and smart ensemble. Shoes should be shiny black and paired with a pair of clean black socks to finish look.

For a formal dress code, a suit with a tie will do just fine. Dark colours like charcoal, navy and grey will best fit the bill. Add a pocket square for that extra touch of elegance, making sure some colour can also be found in the tie.

Cocktail and lounge suit events allow for more creativity, so feel free to add some individuality to your outfit. Lighter coloured suit jackets, sports jackets, fitted shirts — all with no ties — will meet the standard. I like to add a bit of colour when this dress code applies by way of my shirt. I also find it a perfect time to wear loafer shoes with no socks.

A dark pair of good jeans may pass for smart-casual in some social environments, but I would play safe and go for a pair of chinos with a casual shirt (tucked in) or a polo shirt.

Always ensure your belt and shoes match, remember to be a gentleman at all times, and don't forget to sneak $50 into the back of the wallet for the 'maybe' cab ride to get yourself home safe and sound.

First date, checkmate: Dressing for a first date

For most men, the 'First Date' is an emotional roller-coaster of nerves, fear, adrenalin and excitement. These emotions are amplified when you're about to meet the woman you've finally had the courage to ask out. As the saying goes, "You never get a second chance to make a first impression". We all know our behaviour and manners will dictate a great deal as to how the evening will go — and what will get you to a second date. But don't start off on the wrong foot by showing up in clothes that fail to impress.

The way you dress is an extension of your personality. It shows your date a little about yourself and that you respect her enough to make a good impression. It can also make you feel a lot more confident and relaxed, which are the most vital factors in a successful date.

Preparation is key, so choose your outfit the previous day. Don't dress too casually or too formally — go for a smart-casual look. Don't choose an outfit you've never tested out before.

You're not supposed to look different — just a more upmarket version of yourself. Make sure your clothes are neat and clean, as this says a lot about your personal hygiene, self-respect and ability to take care of yourself.

Tailor your outfit to the venue. Don't wear a suit to a rock gig or a rock T-shirt to a five-star restaurant. Clothing colours to consider include black, blue and earthy tones like brown or beige. Unless it is hot and you are going to the beach, stay away from pastel colours. Dress for the weather and dress on the higher end of very smart-casual.

You're probably going to take your jacket off at some point, so make sure your shirt is ironed. Avoid T-shirts with excess slogans, logos or graphics. Jeans and chinos are safe choices. I suggest a quality pair of dark jeans (not distressed or ripped) with a tailored shirt and sports coat. This outfit is smart enough for dinner and casual enough for a drink at a bar. Women notice shoes. Make sure yours are clean and polished.

If you decide to wear jewellery, remember less is more. A nice watch is probably enough.

Arrive on time, don't talk about yourself too much and be interested in her. Ensure you take an interest in her life, job, family and friends. Talking about her dreams and goals, and expressing yours could be a game changer, which she'll respect. Bring up a funny childhood experience as it will show your softer side. Remember to open all doors, pull out her seat and, most importantly, pay the bill no matter what you think of her, as she may have a friend who is Ms Perfect-For-You.

If you want to follow up, do not send a text message. Call her the next day or the day after that. Don't leave it any longer. It's best to call her in the evening straight after work hours. If she answers the phone, thank her for a great night, ask how she is, bring up something you learnt about her from the date, and then schedule a second date. If you reach her voicemail instead, thank her for a great night sounding confident and enthusiastic and ask her to call you back if she has time.

A night to remember: Preparing for a night out

It is part of the Australian culture, to partake in a social drink. It is fun, relaxing and used as a form of bonding when consumed in a sensible, balanced and appropriate way. I remember when I was at the legal drinking age and my Mum said something to me, that to this day still rings in my ears whenever I am enjoying a few quiet drinks, "Pigs don't act like men when they're drunk", meaning gentleman don't get drunk. They are always in control of themselves and the situation. It can be one drink that takes you from cool, to fool. Peer group pressure can be powerful and no guy wants to be known as boring or a stick in the mud. A way to gain the respect of your peers, and be appealing to the females, is to be the guy who is fun, energetic and social but always in control. Be the first to laugh, be spontaneous, interested and open to trying new things. You don't have to be rolling drunk to be that guy.

Watch out for your friends and be the one to diffuse any uncomfortable situations. Be the guy who ensures everyone gets home safely. Your mates will be thankful, as will their parents, partners and colleagues. No female is attracted to guys who loose control of themselves, it is stressful, embarrassing and very uncool and over time, your friends will lose interest in hanging out with you. So you can be the cool guy that everyone respects and admires, a few simple acts could be the difference between being a pig and a man, to use my Mum's analogy. A glass of milk, a meat sandwich, three glasses of water and a sports drink may be the difference between the greatest, fun-filled night of all time, or the all too familiar average night out with unwanted complications.

Preparation is key. Find out where you may be going and take the time to find out about the dress code. Those designer-ripped jeans and expensive sneakers may not be enough for entry. It is a good idea to choose your outfit the day before your night out to allow for any hurdles. Ensure your clothes are all clean and pressed.

Next, wash your hair the night before. Stripping hair of natural oils can leave it flat and lifeless. Hair looks better the day after a shampoo.

On the day, make sure you allow yourself time to get ready. Have a hot shower, scrub your nails, wash and moisturise your face, brush your teeth, use deodorant and apply a masculine cologne. Leave getting dressed to the last minute to avoid unexpected mishaps. Hang your jacket in the car to limit creasing and place mints in the inside pocket with a reserve $50 note for emergencies.

Before getting dressed, prepare a cold meat sandwich for later and drink 500ml of milk to line your stomach. Fill a water bottle and place next to your toothbrush ready to consume before you retire. Place the sports drink next to your bed for when you wake up in the morning, as it will replace lost electrolytes.

The most important rules — be a gentleman, look after your mates and don't mix your drinks.

Mixing business and pleasure:
Tips for social work events

When the silly season approaches, it brings with it the work party. This can be a make or break event for the next 12 months of your employment, or the end of the road if you decide to be a true peanut on the night. A few suggestions should save you from the firing zone and place you at the top of the Christmas tree with projects, pay rises and promotions.

Before the event, determine in advance if partners are invited. A work party is a social gathering and your better half may be a great asset as you work the room. If you don't yet have a better half, this is probably not the best venue for a first date.

Confirm your attendance in advance. Even if you don't feel like attending, make the effort for at least a short time. Determine the dress code; make an impression for the right reasons and stay away from Christmas ties and hats with lights. Make sure you carry money and shout the right people early in the night so they remember. Do not assume everything is free. Don't be first to arrive, or for that matter, too late. Arriving late is a no-no as this will show a lack of interest or that you had something better to do.

Mingle with everyone and their partners early in the night, ensure you include the boss's partner, and remember your manners because they will also. Be an entertaining conversationalist and do not talk work for the entire night. Ask personal questions and be sure to listen, while at the same time using eye contact.

Do not have more than three drinks, eat food with table manners, be a good sport by participating in all activities and watch your dance floor moves.

Here are my top work party tips:

- Do not spoil a good party by staying too late.
- Be mindful of your audience, limit the rude jokes and eliminate foul language.
- Treat hospitality staff with respect, it works both ways and will also limit your chance of receiving a tampered meal.
- Remember to say thank you and goodbye to the right people.
- Be remembered for the right reasons and not be the talk for the next 12 months for acting the class clown.

The wedding planner: Wedding etiquette

Some of life's greatest moments (and life's greatest disasters) can occur at a wedding. A few wedding etiquette tips will ensure you fall into the first category and have you remembered and talked about for the right reasons. Weddings are a great place to network, socialise, meet new people and leave a mark, and this can only be achieved with good behaviour.

It begins once the invitation is received. Be respectful and courteous by sending back an RSVP as soon as possible, as attendance numbers are important. Stragglers at this early stage will leave the bride anxious and she should not have to chase up your reply.

Choose a gift that will be appreciated by both the bride and the groom. Get a group together to buy a bigger gift than each of you would give individually. If you're uncertain about the amount to spend, a rule of thumb is to give at least the equivalent of the cost of your meal, so if you're attending as a couple, double the amount.

An option may be to send the gift before the event — that way you will be seen as excited, prepared and thoughtful.

When considering what to wear, it is far better to be overdressed than underdressed. The invitation will give you an idea of the formality of the occasion. When in doubt, play it safe and wear a jacket and tie. For a more relaxed, non-church wedding on a beach then chinos, linen jacket and a shirt might be acceptable.

Lighter suits are usually suitable for morning and early afternoon ceremonies, with darker colours for late afternoon and evening. Make sure you arrive on time. If, by unforeseen circumstances, you are late, discreetly place yourself at the back. Once at the reception, find your seat and do not move place cards. Seating arrangements were made very carefully for a reason, so no musical chairs.

Introduce yourself early on during the night to both families, paying attention to the elderly. Don't talk during the speeches and look interested — at least pretend to listen while not slouching on the table. Before you leave, be sure to thank the important people, who should definitely include the bride and groom, as well as the people who probably paid for the event, the parents.

Keep the alcohol intake to a moderate level and ensure you employ good table manners when eating. Again, never spoil a good night by staying too late — the good times occur before midnight and the mayhem generally afterwards. In my experience, arguments, fights, getting your kit off, drunken dance moves and regretful hook-ups can be disastrous, so behave!

Budgies vs. boardies: Speedos, shorts or boardies?

While we should avoid covering our banana with a hammock, we should also avoid covering our pole with a tent. As much as the skimpy latex Speedo may turn some ladies off, so will a pair of Bermuda shorts that reach your ankles when wet.

Speedos are the desirable swimwear option only if holidaying in the Mediterranean, swimming the 100 metre final or if you are a qualified lifesaver on duty, complete with red and yellow string cap.

To reduce a farmer's tan on the legs, Speedos can be an option when sunbathing. Just make sure your swimming shorts are within reach for the moment you stand up.

At the other extreme, the long hibiscus-patterned Bermuda shorts have a time and place. That wet, stuck-to your-leg look after swimming doesn't cut it, let alone trying to swim with all that excess fabric. These 35 metres of unnecessary but fabulous material are best kept for fancy dress or watching the Boxing Day test on your couch with a sombrero and your mates (ensuring you do not go outside).

My pick? Place a bet each way during summer and opt for the classic swim short. These are a perfect length and comfortable for all body types, manufactured in a quick drying fabric. A smooth mesh liner is standard, which offers good support for the family jewels and a drawstring offers versatility of fit and snugness when attempting that big bomb off the diving board.

Chapter 5:
Wardrobe Maintenance

Cleaner than squeaky: Washing tips

So far I have given my share of advice and tips on selecting the right clothes — what, when and how to wear them. To get mileage out of our threads, I thought it best to pass on some washing tips (from Mum). To this day no one can launder my clothes like my Mum. The smell, colour and softness can never be equalled, which I put it down to the Melbourne water. I have always observed my dear old Mum's method with great interest to work out her secret formula. This is for the men who are doing their own washing — and for those of you who aren't, you should be helping out with the chores!

To begin the wash cycle, check all pockets for any foreign objects — it's amazing what we put in our pockets. Then check for stains on each item. It is important to remove stains on clothes before washing and drying, so make a pile for anything that needs to be pre-treated, or do it immediately before you forget.

Many of us sort our dirty laundry according to colour. I use these five areas as a general rule of thumb:

- **Whites**
  Whites are separated for a reason — we want them to stay as white for as long as possible. Ensure no bright coloured

items sneak into the mix; this could spell disaster for a white business shirt or new white jocks turning pink with a red sock.

- **Brights**

Brights are colourfast pinks, oranges, yellows, light blues and greens, which can be mixed together for a full load. No red or navy blue here.

- **Reds, dark blues and blacks**

Regardless of age, these colours in the material could bleed onto other fabrics. Play it safe by washing reds separately. Dark blues and blacks can be washed together.

- **Towels**

Towels should be washed separately from clothing because of the amount of lint they produce. If you don't have enough for a complete load, they can be mixed with bed linen.

- **Delicates**

These should be hand washed, or in a machine on a hand-wash or delicate cycle.

Now that's sorted, go ahead and load the machine. Select the water level setting on the machine accordingly, as there must be room for the clothing to circulate freely, otherwise detergent streaks will mark your clothes, which is not a good look.

As far as water temperature goes, all items should be washed in cold water. Cold water works just fine and uses less energy. Detergents and machines have really progressed over the years and almost all colours come out as well in cold water as in warm or hot temperatures.

Follow the instructions on your laundry detergent and use the recommended quantity.

Proper laundry sorting and selecting the correct washing cycle are important keys to a perfect wash, but drying clothes properly can have an equally important part in clothes appearance and longevity.

To help prevent fading and some of the wear and tear associated with the washing and drying phases of laundry, especially for denim jeans and dark pants, turn the clothing inside out before washing and drying. This can reduce fading and pilling of some fabrics, so if you want to prolong the life of your favourites, consider doing this before washing.

No stain, no pain: Stain removal

It doesn't matter how careful you are, rest assured your threads will find a way to attract an unwanted stain at the most inconvenient time. For blokes that aspire to be near-perfect, well-rounded men (huge attraction benefits), learn how to remove the most common stain with products you probably already have at home.

Stain	Action
Red wine	Pour salt onto the stain while it's still fresh, but do not rub. Rinse with warm water after a few minutes. As funny as it sounds, pouring white wine on a red wine stain will help it from setting. Soda water is also an option.

Ink	When ink has leaked from your pen, try spraying hairspray on the stain and rub it in with a dry cloth before washing normally.
Grass stains	If outdoor activities have resulted in grass stains, try sponging some diluted rubbing alcohol on the stain and remove with soapy, warm water. If you can still see remnants of a stain, mix one-part glycerine and two-parts water and cover the stain before it softens.
Motor oil	If your car breaks down and the attempt to fix it has left motor oil on your clothes, place the stain between two paper towels and apply a warm iron to the area. Applying baby powder overnight is also an option.
Deodorant	If a little too much deodorant has stained your shirt at the armpits, soak in white vinegar for 30 minutes before washing. A tablespoon of white vinegar in a measuring cup of water applied with a clean rag will also remove stains from shoes.

Remember to always read the garment label for washing directions and don't forget to take your clothes off the clothesline before it rains.

Iron out the kinks: Ironing tips

I can honestly say ironing would have to be the least favourite and most time consuming chore for most men, but it's necessary if you want to look your best.

Do not expect to be taken seriously or professionally with wrinkled garments; it shows signs of neglectful laziness, which is a tag no man would like to be branded with either professionally or personally.

Ironing know-how was passed on to me by my Nana, who, after Sunday roast would do the ironing while bopping along to Skyhooks when we were all bunkered down watching Countdown.

The process starts with reading the garment label, which will provide you with information about the material. You will find some clothes should not be ironed.

Others have a very low tolerance for heat, so you'll have to iron them on a lower heat setting. Use high heat for cotton and linen. Cotton mixes and wool are ironed on a medium level. Use a low setting for silk, nylon, polyester and similar fabrics.

Ironing shirts

To iron a shirt, begin with the collar. Lay the back of the collar flat and move the pre-heated iron carefully over the surface of the shirt with a few quick strokes. Turn the collar over and do the same to the front.

Place one shoulder over the narrow end of the board and iron from the yoke (the point where the collar meets the arm and the body of the shirt) to the centre of the back. Repeat on the other shoulder.

Next, lay the whole sleeve flat and match the existing creases.

Start ironing at the cuff and work your way to the top of the sleeve. Turn the sleeve over and iron the other side. Repeat the process with the other cuff and sleeve.

Iron both front panels, then flip the shirt over and iron the back. Lastly tackle the panel where the buttons are, taking care to iron between the buttons, as ironing over them can break buttons or scratch your iron's plate.

Once finished, hang your shirts up immediately, ensuring you button the top and centre buttons. Wooden coat hangers make all the difference.

Ironing pants

The best way to iron your pants is to start by turning them inside out. Begin with the top, ironing the circumference of the waistband. Move towards the pockets, ensuring you iron both sides of them. Iron the fly, the pant seams, and then the hems. Follow that order, remembering to use smooth, straight strokes.

Turn the pants so they are the right way out, hook the waistline of the pants around the narrow-shaped end of the board and use the iron to press out the wrinkles of the top-front part of your pants.

Put the pant legs parallel to the board, with both of them headed in the same direction. Iron each leg without damaging the current creases. Hang pants on a wooden hanger immediately while they are still warm.

Three tips to reduce time and get the dry-cleaned look:

- A slightly damp garment is easier to iron and achieves far better results than one that is dry.
- Iron thick fabric on the inside first, then on the outside.

- Use long straight strokes rather than circular strokes. Using a circular motion stretches the fabric and increases the chance of marking.

Pack, stack & rack: Storing your clothes

As the cold, grey days slowly give way to glorious spring sunshine, a clothing change from wool jumpers and coats to cotton polo shirts and pants is sure to take place. With this welcome change, what do we do with our winter attire until next year? Most of us will leave these items hanging in our wardrobe or crammed in the back of the drawer.

Clothes are an expensive and important investment, and will last longer, look better and save you money if stored correctly in the 'off season'.

By following these three simple rules, both you and your garments will be better off for the effort:

- **Clean**
  Your threads are susceptible to bugs, moths, mites and silverfish when they are dirty, so ensure they have one final wash or dry-clean before their vacation.

- **Protect**
  Cedarwood is the easiest and most efficient way of protecting your clothes during storage. The fresh scent repels all unwanted little clothes-destroying guests, while adding a fresh scent to your threads in readiness for the following season. Use cedar blocks for drawers and containers, and

cedar hangers for coats and suits. Storing items in dry, cool, dark, well-ventilated areas will prevent mould and the smell of thrift shop mustiness.

- **Organise**
  A little bit of order will go a long way in mainstreaming and maintaining your wardrobe. Plastic storage crates for jumpers, scarves and hats stored underneath your bed or stacked in a second wardrobe are a great option.

These rules are an integral part of clothing longevity, and will help you stand out from the crowd with dollars left in your wallet.

You have read how I still wear items today purchased years ago, that is because I look after them. I return the favour because my threads look after me.

Packing my dacks: Packing clothes

When I'm travelling for business or pleasure, I need to take the essentials but with space and airline weight considerations packing right and light are the keys.

Spread out everything you'll need for the trip on a bed, then carefully put back at least half of the clothes you've assembled. Less is usually enough, plus it is part of the travelling adventure to buy what you are missing.

Start by placing small valuable items such as sunglasses, mp3 player or jewellery inside a pair of shoes as this will not only protect them, but also save space. Put all liquid toiletry items like cologne, shampoo, conditioner and moisturiser in plastic bags before placing in your toilet bag. Altitude can cause mishaps with containers and this will reduce the chance of your clothes being stained and smelling like a perfume factory.

Turn suit jackets and blazers inside out to protect them from wrinkling. Fold jumpers and knitwear the width of your suitcase or travel bag to prevent bunching. Roll small items such as underwear, shorts, T-shirts and socks. They will act as protection as well as save space.

Packing order should be as follows: start by placing your shoes sole-down at the bottom of your bag or suitcase, followed by jeans and pants folded in half. This will allow a cushion for the more valuable items such as jackets and blazers, which are packed next. Follow this by placing rolled-up underwear, shorts, socks and T-shirts down the sides of your bag or suitcase, and then placing your folded jumpers and knitwear plus toilet bag in last. Pack a few extra plastic bags for dirty laundry.

Once you arrive at your destination hang your jackets, shirts and pants. Use all the available storage space, wardrobes and drawers, at your destination. Place your suitcase or bag away, even if it is for only a few nights as you will enjoy the time more if you are not looking at your luggage!

Keep 'em mean, clean with a sheen: Clean it, store it for longevity

For men who like their threads, the best way to get value for money and longevity out of garments is correct care and storage. When you have invested your hard-earned cash on clothing, following a few simple instructions can add a year or three to their lifespan.

Clothing	Washing Instructions
Jeans	Wash and dry jeans inside out. Only wash jeans after every two to five wears as this will preserve the indigo dye, as well as their shape.
Suits	Dry-clean suits only once a year as the chemicals, solvents and high drying temperatures take their toll. Brush suits to remove lint and dust, not forgetting hidden areas like the neck and armpit areas, which are moth havens. By storing your out-of-season suits in airtight bags you could add five years to their use.
	A clothes steamer is a great investment for cleaning suits but the next best thing is the steam from your morning shower. This will remove creases and the everyday build-up of dirt, sweat and cologne that can discolour a garment.
Shirts	Never get your shirts dry-cleaned, instead machine wash them on a gentle cycle. Once ironed, hang them immediately on wooden hangers with the top button done up to retain the drape and collar shape.

The biggest enemy of your clobber is the moths feeding on keratin, which is a natural protein found in wool, silk and leather. Just because they are not visible, do not think they are not present as they are virtually undetectable when young and at their most potent. Ensuring your clothes are clean prior to putting away is the greatest defence. Vacuuming in key hiding and breeding places like closet corners, along skirting boards, under furniture and at carpet edges will reduce the chances of eaten attire.

Don't be lazy about caring for your clothes. Always take the time to fold and hang them after use and do not leave them in a pile on the floor. Every so often, hang your clothes outside to air them. It may not be the most exciting chore, but wasting money on clothing replacement is not the smartest thing either.

Chapter 6: Grooming

Smooth as silk: The perfect shave

Many men will do it 20,000 times during a lifetime (spending 37.5 days of our lives doing it), each time removing 15,000 to 18,000 hairs totalling over 27 feet in length over a 70-year period.

The 10-minute morning ritual can now be made easier in a three-step process that will leave your skin feeling smooth and rash-free, coupled with a healthy glow.

- **Preparation**

  Always shave after a shower, as steam is the key to opening the pores, which helps raise the whiskers.

  Cleanse with a liquid cleanser that is inexpensive, fragrance-free, and dermatologically tested. While your face is wet, apply sorbolene moisturiser or a five-cent sized dollop of almond oil to the shaving area as this will help eliminate cuts and irritation.

- **Shave**

  Evenly apply shaving cream (not foam) to the moisturised shaving area. Ensure the basin is full with warm water (not too hot), and the blade has been soaking for a few minutes beforehand. Draw the razor along the grain of the beard, starting with the sideburns and cheeks, leaving the thicker stubble areas of the chin and neck more time to soak up the pre-shave and cream application. Always use long, evenly pressured strokes and rinse the blade after every two to four centimetres.

- **Return**
  Rinse your face with cold water to close the pores. As we lose as much skin as hair when shaving, it is important to return moisture and nutrients to the dermis. This is best achieved by applying a non-comedogenic moisturiser (an oil-free one that doesn't block pores) to your wet face, which will help the skin absorb the product quickly and lock extra moisture in.

Shaving Tips

Here are my top shaving tips:
- Every second day, mix bi-carb soda with your liquid cleanser for a cost effective gentle exfoliation.
- If you do happen to get a nick or cut, apply Vaseline and not toilet paper.
- Use single blade shavers for thick beards or three-day growths for less blockage, and twin and triple blades if shaving every day.

Bad breath blues: Treating bad breath

Of the 27 per cent of Australians who suffer from bad breath (halitosis), 19 per cent are men, who spend in excess of $2 billion a year to rid themselves of this unfortunate problem. If you suffer from bad breath, this unwanted and embarrassing issue can affect confidence and self-esteem, which can lead to more serious concerns down the track.

There are two main culprits of bad breath, the first is the build-up of plaque. This causes pockets to develop between the teeth and gums, which then fill with bacteria and food. The second culprit is a dry mouth due to various medications and inhalants.

Good hygiene is by far the best place to start. This includes brushing your teeth and tongue twice a day, combined with flossing and using a mouthwash every night. Research has also shown home remedies are often the best, least harmful and most cost effective approach.

Here are seven tips that, when combined with correct dental care, will help fight the unwelcome problem:

- Add a drop of tea tree oil to your toothpaste before brushing.
- Dilute a ½ tablespoon of apple cider vinegar in a glass of water and gargle for 10 seconds.
- Add a small amount of baking soda to your toothbrush before brushing.
- Chew lemon wedges or drink pineapple juice as this helps pH levels within the saliva.
- Chew mint leaves, parsley or sunflower seeds after a meal.
- Eat plain yoghurt regularly, as it will help fight bacteria.
- Use a tongue scraper to remove bacteria on the tongue, which can cause bad breath. When brushing your tongue with a toothbrush, the bacteria is only stirred and not removed. The best removal practice is by way of a copper tongue scraper which you can buy online or at a health food store.

Hair raising ideas: Hair dos & don'ts

I have no hair on my head, but even so I consider myself an expert on the topic of hair. This includes hairstyle and care, but most importantly, hair dos and don'ts.

In the good old days I had thick, long flowing locks and could walk into any hairdresser and say a sentence which is now just wishful thinking, "Just a little off the side, taper the back, trim the fringe and thin out the top thanks". Unfortunately those days are now long behind me.

Research shows the major causes of hair loss are genes, skin disorders, deficiency in testosterone or iron, ageing, stress and too much hair product. It is normal to lose 50 to 100 hairs a day, so don't be alarmed to see hairs at the bottom of the shower or on the pillow case.

Physical or mental stress can cause hair loss; it often occurs two to three months after the stressful event or period. The reason is that the hair follicles enter the telogen phase prematurely, this is a 'resting' phase which causes new hairs to stop growing, so hair that is shed in not replaced at the normal rate.

Hot oil hair treatments and chemicals used in some hair styling products may cause inflammation of the hair follicle, which can result in scarring of the scalp and hair loss.

So to give you guys who are lucky enough to have an awesome mane a better chance of keeping it, go easy on the care and products. Keep blow-drying to a minimum and pat dry with a towel without rubbing, as being too harsh tends to break hair follicles at the roots.

Use natural styling products, as chemicals in the ingredients will burn your scalp over time. Style your locks with your hands and stay away from bristle brushes, as they tend to pull the hair follicle, which applies unnecessary force to the scalp. As guys have different DNA from our female counterparts, we cannot withstand the treatment and products they can endure.

Once you see your hair receding at the front or the bullseye at the back of your head, don't be afraid to get some advice from hair loss professionals, as today's methods and technology are so advanced. If you're hair starts thinning don't do the comb-over, as long hair will only accentuate the problem; a closer crop will maximise coverage. Above all, look after yourself with the tips in this chapter and try not to stress.

Scary hairy: Removing unwanted hair

I am sure, along with a large percentage of men, that the best invention for men's grooming would be a 'hair transfer'. Imagine waking up each morning and instead of washing those precious whiskers from the daily shave down the drain, trimming those nose and ear hairs or viewing that mohair jumper that is starting to form on your shoulders and back, if those hairs were instead transferred to the top of your head. Hey presto! No bald guys, no grizzly bears at the beach, and all the while it would improve unemployment by creating more hairdressing salons!

Unfortunately, as we all know this is not possible, so it's best we remove those little follicles in all those unwanted places by the least painful, practical and long-lasting method we can.

There are four common options on offer (not including the timeless tweezers to just rip it out):

- **Shaving**
This is the most common method of hair removal, which can be applied to most areas (but consider carefully for sensitive areas). As stated previously, preparation is the key to reducing rashes and ingrown hairs. Also remember that when you shave the hair feels prickly when it grows back, so give serious thought to eyebrows, shoulders and your back.

- **Waxing**
This involves spreading hot wax onto the desired area, then applying a strip of cloth or muslin onto the wax, rubbing it and ripping off the strip in one motion — wax, hair, root and all. The process can be painful, particularly on areas with thinner skin. Just ensure you are ready. No pain, no gain!

- **Laser treatment**
Laser treatment involves a laser beam directed at the hair follicles, which kills them and offers a permanent reduction in hair quantity. As it is the most effective and lasting hair removal procedure, it is the most expensive. In saying this, other treatments are frequent and add up over time.

- **Hair removal creams**
These can be your best option if you don't have the budget or if you dread the pain involved in the waxing process. Pharmacies and supermarkets now provide a good selection of creams ready for home use.

It's worth taking the time to choose your option carefully, as woman would rather go to the zoo to see hairy creatures than the bedroom!

Helping hands & feet: Hand & feet care

Your hands and feet are the hardest working parts of your body. The 52 bones of a pair of feet are 25 per cent of the body's total number of bones. Together with 33 joints, 107 ligaments and 19 muscles of each foot, they support your weight and carry you around.

Over the course of the day there are not many tasks that don't include your hands, so it's about time we started looking after these neglected portions of our body.

Typical foot problems include sores, athlete's foot, cuts, ingrown toenails, bunions and calluses . The best preventative measures start with the correctly-sized selection of shoes and socks. As basic as this sounds, incorrect footwear is the largest cause of feet problems.

Wash your feet daily and rinse and dry thoroughly, especially between the toes. Use talc powder for the best results. Nails should be trimmed straight and not too near the nail bed in order to prevent infections. Avoid digging out and cutting at corners; this could result in painful ingrown toe nails.

Many people will notice your hands straight away; they are the most exposed part of the body. Protection from the elements is the best measure and will help reduce age and/or liver spots (those brown spots that appear on your hands as you get older). Get in the habit of applying sunscreen every day and clip your nails at least once a week.

For those men who have a partner, give her a massage with oil while watching TV — this will not only get you in the good books, but it will moisturise your hands at the same time. For guys without a partner, you can apply oil to your feet before you go to bed!

Clean & dry up: The importance of drying yourself

A survey by Men's Health magazine of married and single women revealed the biggest turn off for them is unhygienic and unclean men, so men it's time to clean (and dry) up your act.

The usual shower and deodorant ritual for us hairy, sweaty beasts is not enough, as new test show men have more areas in which bacteria is trapped. The biggest mistake made is not drying off properly in those all important areas after a shower, which creates a bacterial breeding ground. No matter how much soap and scrubbing we do, if not adequately dry under those hairy armpits and in the groin region we are a walking, infested breeding gound for bacteria; a scientist's dream maybe but a female's nightmare.

Not drying off properly will also cause wet undergarments and clothing and a musty smell, which no cologne will overpower. The garment drying process without air and sunshine takes on average six to nine hours, and staining will also make clothes unwearable. Women notice everything with male hygiene and grooming maintenance, and the five most noticeable things are smell, hair, nails, skin and teeth.

So my tip is after you have shampooed and conditioned your locks, washed your important body parts, scrubbed your nails and washed your face, reach for a big, thick, clean towel and dry yourself like never before. Then dry again before brushing your teeth, then rinse with mouthwash, apply moisturiser and use a splash of cologne. You will now be an irresistible, dry, sweet-smelling Adonis.

Facial furring: Facial hair to suit your face

We all grow it, most of us shave it off, but if you are wanting a change this might be your answer. By selecting the right facial hairstyle you can emphasise your best features and hide your worst flaws. On the other end of the scale, you can also highlight those flaws by wearing the wrong look.

If you want a change in the way of some designer stubble, here are the facial hair styles best suited to the four most common face types:

- **Face type: square**
  Men with square faces should lean towards styles that make their mug appear less box-like and more long and slender. The best way to achieve this is a light all-over beard that is clipped every other day. Pay more attention to the Adam's apple area and around the mouth for a clean look.

- **Face type: round**
  Round faces are best suited to facial hairstyles that make their faces look oval and elongated. To achieve this, sport a circle beard. A circle beard is a moustache that continues along the sides of the mouth and meets the hair on the chin, but no side burns. Shave your jaw and neck every day, and use clippers every three to four days on your stylised circle beard.

- **Face type: rectangle**
  A beard will help men with oblong faces, as it will help balance their features by way of shortening the face length. Clipper your beard every three to five days and blade-shave your neckline to reduce looking like Grizzly Adams.

- **Face type: triangle**
Triangular-shaped faces usually have pointy chins, and the best way to change this shape is by adding weight along the jawline and chin. A fuller beard is perfect for this. Clipper once a week for a respectable look and also tidy up the Adam's apple with a blade.

Men lucky enough to have an oval shaped face can get away with anything. Remember it is facial hair and grows back so don't be afraid to experiment for a different look. There is a reason, however, that 'Movember' only goes for a month and it's best we all keep it that way.

Everybody sweat now: Sweating tips

Sweating is a natural process, but when the bad odour and armpit hoops also join the party, alarm bells start ringing. Added to this, the damage that sweat does to clothes can be non-repairable, so a few tips will help you save some hard-earned money along the way.

Begin with a chemical free, non-comedogenic, low fragrance antiperspirant deodorant to start the day. If your problem is a real concern, use a rock crystal as these crystals naturally protect against bacteria and therefore neutralise odour from sweat. They can be found at health food stores.

You can also apply rock crystal to any part of your body that tends to sweat a lot such as the spine area of your back, inner thighs and lower neck.

Your antiperspirant needs to come in contact with your skin

in order to work. A problem will occur when your armpit hair becomes exceedingly long, and therefore acts as an obstacle between the product and your skin. I am not suggesting an underarm wax, but a subtle trim with scissors will help.

Wearing fabrics like cotton, silk or linen instead of polyester or other synthetics and blended fabrics will also help. Natural fibres allow your skin to breathe more, meaning you'll sweat less and look cool.

If those dreaded armpit rings are a problem, layering can actually help sweat-proof your clothes. Your best bet is to layer with a sports undershirt underneath a T-shirt. When you have to wear a dress shirt, choose a sports undershirt in white that won't be too noticeable. Sports clothes are specifically designed to keep moisture away from your body, and they also dry quickly, so you'll never feel like you're soaking in sweat.

When cleaning your shirts, soak them in cold water and apply a stain remover to the armpits. To achieve the best results and really get stains out, turn your shirt inside out and apply the stain remover to the inside of your shirt. This works better than applying it to the outside of your shirt because you're trying to lift the stain out of the fabric, not rub it further into the fibres.

Leave the product on for a few minutes and launder your shirt as soon as possible, or at least rinse it in ice-cold water again. If your shirt is white, bleach it every now and again. For heavier garments such as suit jackets, hang them outside overnight to refresh them. No sweat!

Wake up & smell the roses: Choosing the right scent

In 1987 whilst at Singapore airport in the duty-free store I discovered Chanel ANTAEUS as my perfect scent and have used it ever since.

A commonly asked question from my clients now is, "What cologne should I buy?" Like art and wine, cologne is very subjective and a number of factors should be considered before handing over your hard-earned cash and running the risk of smelling like the Botanic Gardens or the local dump.

The two most important factors in your decision are skin type and lifestyle. When I say 'skin type' you can fall into one of two categories: oily or dry skin.

Oily skin enhances and amplifies your cologne and responds best to a lighter, citrus-based scent. These elements help to balance out the stronger natural odours your skin is producing. Choose more airy-based scents for a fresher, crisper smell.

Dry or sensitive skin does not hold a scent for as long as oily skin, as cologne needs something to adhere to. You would think applying more is the answer, but this is not the case. Instead, try heavier or thicker scents with undertones of tobacco and musk; these have a greater presence and will stay with you longer.

Consider your lifestyle when deciding on your next smell-good. For example, are you big on spicy foods? Are you a big drinker? Do you smoke? What you ingest comes to the surface of your skin in perspiration and blended with the wrong cologne might not have you smelling like you think.

When in the store, apply cologne to scent cards, as this will give you the opportunity to individualise each cologne. A good tip is to smell coffee beans in between. Once you have chosen a scent, let it sit for a few minutes and then smell the card again. A strong scent will linger too long and become offensive. The right scent will dissipate and settle into a nice pleasant aroma.

Apply your new signature scent to behind your ears, the glandular points on your neck and/or your inner wrists, as these three body locations carry the aroma longer.

All year, round & round: Winter routine

The harsh winter climate increases the amount of time spent indoors and the area most affected is our skin. Lack of sunshine and fresh air, exposure to artificial and recycled heating methods coupled with strong, cool drying winds outside can age us prematurely, just like to much sun, if we don't take care.

A simple effective daily routine can help you avoid looking pale and unhealthy. Forget the macho mindset and the stigma once associated with a men's skincare routine — what was once a minority is now a majority, so conform and reap the benefits by putting those outdated ideas about men not using moisturiser behind you.

Products once only available from speciality shops are now available in supermarket and chemist shelving; old school brands like Gillette and Brut now offer a complete range of everything you need.

Follow this swift and simple two-minute routine, guaranteed to make you look and feel great.

If you do nothing else, cleansing is the single most important thing you can do for your face, and should be the basis of your skincare routine. Typically, men's skin has large pores and very active sebaceous glands. While these glands are critical for keeping the skin naturally moist, they can often produce too much sebum, leaving your skin feeling greasier than an oil slick. Neglecting to wash away the excess oil and dirt can clog pores, which leaves the skin prone to breakouts.

A cleanser washes away oil and dirt on the surface, but what about all that nasty stuff deep down in your pores? That's where exfoliation should be part of your ritual twice a week; it will help displace debris normal cleansing can't. A good scrub should have granules to help eliminate dry skin associated with cooler conditions, while also reducing pore clogging and dirt build-up.

It is important to replenish, feed and protect your face in the colder months, so moisturise and ensure SPF30 is present in your product. This will add a shield to all the elements, while replenishing and feeding lost natural oils, which will help prevent the skin from drying out and becoming white and flaky.

An effective lip balm is a must; unkissable lips are not a good look. As the skin on your lips is incredibly thin and lack oil glands, they are prone to dryness and cracking when exposed to the elements. I'm an old-school kind of guy that likes to use tried and tested products. Chapstick is my preference; it's been around since the late 1800s and is a product that is available worldwide. I also prefer the method of a stick application as I think applying product with my fingers is unhygienic when hand-washing facilities are not available.

Stranger than fiction:
Grooming myths & old wives' tales

The tales told by our parents to stop us doing embarrassing things in our youth, like pulling funny faces or picking our noses, was often a predicted drastic outcome that would ensure the end to such behaviours! If the wind changed direction, our face would be permanently cross-eyed. If we continued picking our nose, our eyes would fall out.

Myths and misconceptions have always been around and men's grooming is no exception. I have put together the top three myths I have heard in my time and must confess, believed them for a minute or two — plus a couple that are actually true.

Top Grooming Myths

I think these are the top grooming myths:

- **Toothpaste helps acne (False)**
  I was a sucker for this one in my teens. As teenagers we try anything, and Mr Colgate's profit margins must have increased tenfold on the back of this. There is not one ingredient in toothpaste that would remotely cure or help control the dreaded zit.

- **Only use sunscreen in summer (False)**
  This is a common misconception and a very costly one to your skin. The sun of today is different to decades ago, and with that comes the need for extra protection. It is best to apply a facial sunscreen all year round.

- **Washing your face with body soap will do (False)**
  It is called 'body soap' for a reason as it will leave your body clean, but as your pores differ on your face, you will be left with irritated, dry skin with constant use. Buy a facial cleanser, apply your SPF and reap the rewards.

- **Shave after a shower for a closer shave (True)**
  Shaving after a shower will soften your beard and open your pores, which will give a closer, comfortable and less irritated shave.

- **Teabags help tired and puffy eyes (True)**
  The mix of caffeine and antioxidants from a pre-used morning cup of tea will help reduce puffiness and redness, and bring tired eyes to life. Just make sure the teabag has cooled.

Chapter 7:
The Keys to Confidence

You da man: The importance of confidence

One common trait which successful men from all walks of life have, including elite athletes, successful businessman and even Joe the plumber, is confidence — the belief in oneself and one's power and abilities.

We all have days when we have the George Clooney -swagger and nothing will faze us. Then there are those days when you are more like 'Raj' from Big Bang Theory with little confidence with women.

We all need and love the feeling of confidence for different reasons. The key is to find out where you need to improve, and then go out and believe in your abilities, talents, experience, look and personality. When you have confidence and belief in yourself, life is more fun, fulfilling and enjoyable.

When the 'Raj' days hit you, ensure you surround yourself with good, positive people. Family and friends will recognise your ups and downs, and offer support and encouragement if required.

Always be open-minded and well-rounded, as the art of conversation is a great stimulus and connector to socialise with people on all levels. Make the time to partake in and enjoy the things you excel at, as doing the things you are good at brings a sense of importance and satisfaction.

We all judge people on first impressions and body language is often the first sign in this process. It's because our mannerisms, poses and postures are a great source of information. They reflect our mood and our confidence level. As stated by the George/Raj example, how you stand and walk sends a message. At a glance, most people can discern if we're apprehensive or outgoing, relaxed or aggressive, fun or boring, happy or sad.

In order to be viewed as a self-assured and confident person, a few things to remember are:

- Stand tall and proud.
- Walk with purpose.
- Look ahead, not down.
- Don't cross your arms.
- Avoid putting your hands in your pockets.
- Don't fidget.

More often than not, the way you perceive yourself will be the way others think of you also, so let's all be cool like Steve McQueen, handsome like Brad Pitt and charming like George Clooney.

Ladies and gentleman: Being a gentleman

Before you understand how to be cool in these modern times, you need to know what people, and more so woman, expect from a man and what you can do to be that man. Dressing and looking the part only plays a very small piece in the jigsaw of 'cool'. Actions are long remembered and even if you look a million dollars, if you don't act like a million dollars, you're only worth small change, if anything at all.

We all know some things change and evolve at a rapid rate; it's the world we live in. But some things are best thought, spoken and practiced how they once were. The most important ingredients to the complete 'cool' puzzle are truth, loyalty and courtesy.

Don't look at these traits as old fashioned or out-dated, they are the foundations of what it takes to be cool. These traits don't need to change just because we're in the 21st century, because, let's face it — there are some things that were done yesteryear that were way cooler than what we do today.

Truth provides the foundation of any relationship, be true to yourself and others. Loyalty denotes a relationship that is based on truth and commitment. Courtesy provides the means for cordial and meaningful relationships.

Setting the right example with these three traits sends a message, which is far more powerful than any suit or designer outfit.

Once the foundation has been laid, your well on your way to being a cool, confident, respectful, generous and open-minded guy that men will envy and women will greatly admire. Make the time to be a better person by way of action, appearance and beliefs.

Start today by holding open the door for people, especially when they are carrying heavy things or are not as physically fit as you are. Share your umbrella, even if that means you get wet for a few seconds. Give your coat to a woman when she's cold, draping it over her shoulders and making sure she's warm. Compliment in a sincere and truthful way.

Be nice to your girlfriend's friends. It's one thing to be good to your girlfriend; it's a whole new level to be nice to her friends. Leave little notes around for her to find. When the waiter comes, asking her what she'd like and letting her order first. Sending a little message to make sure she got home all right. But keep the text messages, pictures, emails, and any other exchanges that happen between you just that — between the two of you. No bragging to friends.

Bring her coffee or tea in the morning. It doesn't have to be a regular thing it's a small gesture that shows a lot of kindness. Give flowers, no need to wait for a special occasion. Send something every now and again to her office. Stand up for her if she's being spoken to aggressively. Call when you say you are going to call. Be kind and respectful to wait staff when dining out together. Ask her to dance. Remember special days. Walk on the outside of the footpath.

All these actions are easy, thoughtful and long remembered. Be known as the perfect guy in every way: honest, thoughtful, sincere, and strong. Mr Cool.

Unfortunately something I've noticed lacking in today's world is sincere gratitude and chivalry. It was only a generation ago that a man was measured by his manners and etiquette.

Are we turning into a generation of expecting, ungrateful, dissatisfied, spoilt, classless dudes only interested in self-gratification? Well guys, it's time to get back to some of the good old-fashioned manners our parents and grandparents valued.

One particular gripe of mine is the lack of gratitude I see in receiving gifts. It seems as though the thought of giving is no longer relevant and has been overtaken by the size and cost of the gift. I experienced this firsthand at Christmas recently when giving a fun gift to someone (which was not required as it was a Kris Kringle). The recipient did not say 'thank you', let alone 'Merry Christmas'. The look of disappointment was so obvious once it was unwrapped that I had to turn away from embarrassment. No, it was not an expensive gift and obviously so, but surely the thought and effort taken to decide what to buy, purchase, wrap and give it in good faith must be acknowledged in some way?

It is so easy to say thank you. We can say it in person, over the phone, via text or email, and for a greater impact, write a card and post it. This last, often forgotten deed says so much more than electronically abbreviating a three-second message and pushing 'send'.

Let's not be seen as wimpy robots, but have a go at looking like a suave, well-mannered and charming James Bond-type gentlemen.

Tips to being a gentleman

These are my tips to being a suave gentleman:

- Be grateful and give acknowledgement.
- Display good manners by listening more and talking less.
- Don't groom yourself in public, look at your watch or flaunt your riches.
- Maintain eye contact, shake hands firmly and be punctual.
- Never talk with your mouth full or use the serviette as a hanky or face towel.
- When in the presence of women, open doors, give up your seat, help her with her coat and ask her if she needs anything. Let me assure you, these gentlemanly virtues are still highly valued by women!

Scent of a woman: Buying her a gift

There is no better way to show our appreciation to the beautiful women in our life than to take the time and effort to select the right perfume. Your thoughtful, creative, personal and distinctive decision shows complete confidence, elegance and old fashioned values, which will be acknowledged and rewarded.

When selecting the right scent for your loved one it will help to realise there some scents more suitable to day time wear, and others which are more suitable to evening. Fruity, floral, citrus and fresh green notes are good considerations for day. They tend to be brighter, dewy and crisp. Musks, woods (cedar wood, sandalwood), suede notes and vanilla are usually used for evening application. A general rule of thumb is that fruity floral fragrances seem to resonate more with younger women (18 to 30). For women over 40 it is more about stronger floral, oriental or creamy, woody scents.

They say that a man's biggest mistake when selecting a perfume is selecting it because they like the way it smells on someone else. That is a huge mistake. Odds are more than likely it will not smell the same on the woman you are buying it for. Everybody has different chemistry, hence the warmth of the skin, eating habits and what other skincare products are used all play a role in how a fragrance will smell on an individual's skin.

Perfumes will fall under three categories: classic, delicate and sensual. A classic perfume is best given to a female when you are unsure of her personality or would like to play it safe. (One would hope this would not apply to your mum or wife). A delicate perfume best suits a sophisticated and feminine woman. If you are buying a perfume for a bold and confident woman who is also passionate towards others, get her the sensual perfume.

Research your beauties. Be observant and in tune to what the woman you are buying for likes and dislikes. What does she wear now, which scents does she like and what best sums up her personality and style?

Specialty perfume shops and department stores can offer a breadth of advice, but knowing the basic likes and dislikes of who you are shopping for will help you choose a scent they will adore and think of you every time it is applied. Now that has got to be good.

Romancing the stone: Female etiquette

The advice that has served me best over the years is, 'Respect and romance a woman and reap the rewards'.

Being a romantic has nothing to do with losing your blokey image or macho masculinity. As it is the strong, smart and classy guy who understands and values the love of a good woman. It is also the open-minded contemporary man who will go to any effort to make his woman feel like the most important and beautiful woman on earth.

This does not mean buying expensive gifts, as the poorest man alive can have the happiest partner in the world. One of the most thoughtful gifts you can give a woman is your time and attention. This means talking, and more importantly, listening.

Tell her at every opportunity how beautiful she is. Make sure to do this not only when she is at her best, that is, when she is all dressed up and happy, but more importantly, when she feels at her worst.

Listen to her and don't interrupt, tune out or try to 'fix' her problems. Offer advice when asked, but be sympathetic. By keeping each other informed and having time to talk together, you will keep the relationship healthy, close and happy.

Touch is also important — and it's free. A hug, kiss or squeeze is a great form of expression and great for her ego; it never goes unnoticed.

Laughter and humour is the key to any good time, so be sure to use your sense of humour. Be silly, play pranks and do impersonations at odd times because to see a woman laugh is one of life's great joys.

Spontaneity is also a winner. Doing things when least expected has far greater impact than knowing when something is going to happen. Arrange a date night and surprise her. None of this is rocket science guys, it is just the old adage of 'happy wife, happy life'.

Start at the end & begin at the start: Starting & ending the day

Fortunately, every day we wake to a new beginning, never knowing what may lie ahead in these often challenging hours before it ends and starts all over again. I have found that routine is the best way of forming good habits. To help make this easier I built awareness around my bad habits by writing a list of pros and cons. The biggest factor in breaking a habit is having proper awareness around it in the first place.

Writing another list of how my life would improve without the habit was also helpful in the process. Having this checklist ensured responsibility and provided something to answer to. I was lucky growing up in a sporting family with my brothers playing AFL, witnessing firsthand their discipline, good habits and the best way to achieve it. A healthy body and mind are one of life's great treasures and the only person who can do this for you is yourself.

To keep you on the top of your game both mentally and physically,

I have put together my morning and nightly ritual. Stick your toe in the water first, and by that I mean try to incorporate one of the morning and nightly tasks for a week and then over time add more. Be realistic with your goals and efforts and most importantly be honest with yourself. Change is often difficult but when the by-product is good health, a positive outlook, a calm soul and an energetic being, the time and effort will definitely be worth it.

The two most important hours of the day to achieve this awesome feeling are the first and last hour of each day.

Morning

Early bird: As much as we all love sleep, I find setting the alarm 30 minutes earlier than usual is the best way to maintain a calm start to the day. Running late first thing in the morning is the start of a harder than usual day ahead. The way you spend the first hour of the day often sets your mood, energy and temperament for the remainder of the day. To begin, try with setting the alarm 10 minutes earlier for the first week, which is enough to tick it off the list.

Move the body: Often the hardest steps of the day are the first two: getting out of bed and moving your body. However, your body will love you if you make the effort to complete some form of exercise first thing in the morning. It is the best way to keep your body lean and trim, as you are burning fat residuals (people who exercise later in the day have to do that little extra bit of work). It will also help with your energy levels and leave your mind in the most perfect state ready to tackle anything with a positive 'can do' attitude. I found the key was to set out my exercise attire the night before, that's shoes and all, right at the end of the bed. Following a program and setting a few realistic goals are also useful tools.

Fuel: Take the time to have a healthy breakfast, as it sets you up for the whole day. Options are plentiful so make the effort to stock the cupboards with good cereals, breads and fruit. Experiment with smoothies and omelettes, taking notice of what fruits and vegetables are in season. Again, I pull it out and set up the night before and doing this also helps with product stock levels and if I need to I go shopping that night. I like ease and convenience so I keep the cooked breakfasts for the weekend.

The three sss: Shave, Scent and Sunscreen

Allow the time to have a good shower and shave properly, as it will give you a more healthy appearance and indicate that you care about your appearance. I love this time, as it is a reward for the previous hour. Looking in the mirror when you are full of beans and feeling six feet four is the perfect start to a great day!

Always shower first to allow the beard to soften for a closer more comfortable shave. No matter what time of year, moisturise your skin with a SPF30. We all know what damage UV rays cause but a moisturizer with SPF30 will also add protection to other harmful pollutants which are present all year round.

Switch and experiment with a new cologne every few months, as the people around you will appreciate the change. Use seasons as a guide and choose more woody and earthy fragrances for cooler climates and more floral for warmer weather. I find the feeling of cleanliness and freshness a little confidence pill that gives me an I-can-take-on-anything feeling.

Night

This time of day is often the hardest to keep a routine due to family, work and social commitments but I always find that if by following my little routine below means 45 minutes less sleep, it is worth it.

Electronic-less: I know it can be difficult, but stay away from all electronic gadgets the last hour before bed, which includes TV. A recent study by the Medical Journal of Australia stated a particular energy emitted from electronic devices plays havoc with a hormone beneficial for a good night sleep. I find reading the day's newspaper and catching up on my football news the best. Choose something irrelevant to work so you can escape completely and achieve a clear mind for that perfect night's sleep.

Stretch: This is the secret for me. When it is quiet and calm, the kids are safely tucked away then my body gets an oil change and grease. Take a minute to think of the positions your body goes through over the day. Stretching for ten minutes will not only relax you, but also elongate your muscles providing a leaner, more toned appearance. Dip that toe and start off gently as there are no prizes for elastic man. As time goes by increase the stretches and become more adventurous in your poses and use different muscle groups. It was only a few years ago I could not touch my toes. The by-product is great posture and a clear head.

Prepare: Take the time to prepare for the following day by choosing and laying out the clothes you plan to wear, and whilst you're doing this, put the exercise gear by the bed. This will give you more time in the morning and will help you make better decisions than a mad-rush morning scram. Pack a lunch as it will not only save you time and money, but you will reap the rewards for fuelling your body with left-overs or healthy homemade options instead of processed alternatives. I know you would rather be doing something more relaxing as you are tired from the day's events but making the effort and taking the time is well worth it.

Pamper: Reward time again. Use the end of the day for a grooming ritual and practise proper hygiene routines. Don't just brush your teeth, but take the time to also floss and use a mouthwash. This will provide strong healthy teeth, gums and a killer smile. It will also help with the morning (bad) breath. Wash and moisturise your face, taking the time to find a product that suits your skin type. Twice a week take the time for an Epsom salts bath (a ritual for me). It will not only relax your weary muscles but also helps draw out any impurities and toxins within the body.

There it is guys, the 8-step routine to start and finish your day on the right foot. I know some of you will use the excuse of 'not having enough time', but try and follow this the best you can. Time is one of life's precious commodities and there is only 24-hours in a day, but believe me, you can make time. It is definitely worth the effort, as feeling great is precious commodity.

On your marks, get set, go!:
Never too late to feel good

Life can be busy and stressful but that should not be the excuse for not making yourself a better, happier and healthier person through small changes and new experiences. The feeling of accomplishment is a great way to enhance your confidence and self-esteem. However, as we grow older, the fear of failure can limit us from trying new things. It is never too late for change and only one person is capable of making this happen, you.

Take small steps to begin the process, as the old saying goes, 'from little things big things grow'.

Looking back on my life I have compiled a list of 'things to do' which were instrumental and beneficial for me to experience that wonderful feeling of achievement, self-worth and increased confidence.

Here is my 'to do' list to creating a sense of accomplishment:

- **Build something**
  It gives you a great sense of accomplishment when you finish a project.

- **Do yoga**
  This creates a great connection between body and mind. You will have more energy, and at the same time look and feel better too.

- **Read a book**
  Give the TV a miss twice a week and find a good book (there are plenty out there).

- **Get a check-up**
  Make an appointment for a visit to the doctor to confirm that everything is working the way it should be.

- **$20 a week**
  Put aside this amount each week and buy yourself something special this time next year.

- **Learn to cook**
  There's no better way to enjoy your fruits of labour, let alone impress anyone and everyone.

- **Help someone**
  The best way to feel better about yourself is by helping someone else who needs a hand.

It is your life, so be looked upon and remembered as someone who lived life to the fullest and experienced new things and change with open arms. You owe it to yourself and your loved ones.

It's all in the plan, Stan: Planning your time

Time is a commodity we all wish we had more of. It seems that as we get a little older this valuable resource becomes scarcer.

As kids, the only relevant 'time' was bedtime, then later as singles we think how strapped for time we are with such a hectic social calendar. It seems only when we become parents can we truly appreciate how much time we used to have. It appears that today, time and excuses go hand in hand. Don't have time to exercise, eat properly, catch up with family and friends, fix the tap, and remove the rubbish— the list goes on.

With only 24-hours in a day, the only way to have enough time is time management. All successful people have had enough time to achieve and accomplish goals because they have planned, prioritised and been productive.

Time Management Tips

- **Plan your day**
  Planning your day can help you accomplish more and help you feel more in control of your life. Write a to-do list (daily, weekly and monthly), putting the most important tasks at the top. Set the alarm 30 minutes early, as this is the ideal time to exercise, stretch and to think about the day ahead. Be mindful of what you have ahead, as multi-tasking can add

time to the 'time bank'. Buy food when walking past the shop, pay the bill on the way to lunch — planning ahead is the key. Be punctual at all times, as 10 minutes late will turn the rest of the day upside down.

- **Prioritise**

  Prioritising tasks will ensure you spend your time and energy wisely. Don't make the mistake of thinking that doing everything will give you time at the end of the day or at the end of the week. Some things have to be done now but some tasks can be put on the back burner — just ensure they remain on the weekly or monthly list. As hard as it may be, learn to say 'no' sometimes.

- **Productivity**

  Use your time wisely. It is one of the few things we get for free, but we can never have it back. A very successful and happy man once said to me, "There are 24-hours in a day. Sleep eight, work eight and live eight the way you want to, but make sure you learn and achieve at least one thing a day".

Straight as an arrow: The benefits of good posture

No matter what brand of clothes you wear and how much you spend, if you do not have the correct posture, you will look like the Hunchback of Notre Dame wearing a two-man tent.

In today's lifestyle with computers, big screen TVs and long commute times, we can find ourselves in awkward sitting positions for long periods of time.

It's time to straighten up, stand tall, square your shoulders and hold your head up high. It's remarkable how good posture can change your outlook, stress levels and how people view you. Good posture starts with three activities we do all day, every day: standing, sitting and sleeping.

When standing tall and erect, your ears, shoulders, hips, knees and ankles should make one straight line. Relax your shoulders and slightly bend your knees — you don't want to look and move like a stormtrooper from Star Wars. If you're in a situation where you are required to stand for a long period of time, ensure you shift your weight and position every so often.

When seated, make sure you sit with your hips as far against the back of the chair as possible and keep your knees at hip level while your spine runs firmly along the back of the chair. If your back is not getting the necessary support from the back of the chair, try placing a small pillow or a rolled up towel to support your lower back. When you sit at a desk, make sure it is at elbow height. If you're looking at a computer screen, tilt it upwards so you are looking slightly up instead of down, which will create a natural curve in the spine.

The same principles apply when driving. Place your hips as far back in the seat as possible while holding the steering wheel with your elbows slightly bent.

Try to avoid sleeping on your stomach. Sleeping on your back or side on a firm mattress will have you waking up without a twisted spine. Of course I'm sure I don't have to mention that when bending down, ensure you bend your knees and not your waist!

With good posture the benefits are astounding. You'll not only feel more energetic and vibrant, but look thinner, stronger, taller and more sure of yourself.

The Midas touch: Stress relief

If I said for a dollar a day you could reduce anxiety, enhance sleep quality, have more energy and create better posture, all while feeling five years younger and with no side effects, do you think it would be a good investment? Absolutely!

All this can be achieved by having a massage every three months. Most people would agree a massage makes them feel good, but many probably don't realise exactly how good a regular massage is for their overall health.

Massage increases the blood's oxygen capacity by 10 to 15 per cent, balances the nervous system by soothing or stimulating it, increases production of gastric juices, saliva and urine, and increases excretion of nitrogen, inorganic phosphorus and sodium chloride, which in turn increases your metabolic rate.

Levels of stress hormones like adrenalin, cortisol and norepinephrine are also reduced. As men we are sometimes reluctant to look after ourselves properly and break from the old school attitude of "Nah, I'm all right" and ignore our health, as we want to be seen as strong and invincible to our peers.

We are also reluctant at times to move from our fathers 'old ways' to a new open-minded approach to our health and wellbeing. Walking into a massage/beauty therapy premises today is not as daunting as you would think. All of these benefits are a sure way to feel great, enhance your relationships and improve your health, and all for around a buck a day. A quarterly massage is the key for a healthier tomorrow. Relax and enjoy!

Shake, shake, shake: The gentleman's handshake

My 85-year-old grandfather has been teaching my five-year-old son the importance of a good, firm, manly handshake. It's not just about this tradition as a greeting, but the impression it portrays.

To receive a handshake from a man the power of a wet fish is not the right way to start proceedings. As men, we have all experienced different handshakes in our time. The memorable ones seem to be for the wrong reason: too soft, too wet, too timid or too firm.

A soft handshake gives a first impression of lack of confidence and interest with no masculinity, which is not the ideal start. Hold the hand with as much force as you hold a stubby, not a baby chicken.

A wet handshake is a sure sign of nerves and inferior social skills. If you suffer from this, carry a hanky and wipe your hands beforehand, and keep your hands open instead of in a fist.

A timid handshake is from the guy who only grabs four fingers towards the tips. If this does happen to you, pretend you didn't hear his name and shake again, but this time properly and make sure he knows it.

The too-firm handshake automatically says ego problems with too much testosterone. There is no need to bring the he-man tough guy to the greeting. It is not a competition of strength.

A handshake says a lot about your confidence, character and security with oneself, or lack thereof. The perfect etiquette handshake is as follows:

- Ensure you are standing straight and use eye contact and a smile.
- Extend your right hand with fingers lightly spread and elbow slightly bent, while leaning a little toward the other person.
- Take the other person's hand firmly and fairly: the correct pressure is similar to holding a golf club ready to swing.

- Release the hand after two to four pumps.

It is said you can decode a person by his handshake so make this forgotten gentlemanly art the right code for you.

The 20 Life Rules

Your 'brand' is what people think of you when they see and meet you. As guys, we are our own brand. As strange as you may think that sounds, we are walking, living individual brands. We have spent years with people easily judging our brand on first visual impressions, and then as time goes on, our personality.

I've given you the guidance, instruction and direction in this book to make your brand a stylish, modern, respectful and lasting one. Below is my 20-life rule list that is the icing on the cake to make your brand 'cool'.

I've compiled this list over the years from watching and listening intently to the beautiful and fascinating people around me. By trying to treat and respect people from all walks of life the same and by being true to myself, I've come to regard mistakes as part of the journey, so I'm no longer afraid of failure. Here are a few things I've learned and observed about the world we live in:

- The best success is living the life you want for yourself and your family.
- Be open-minded and try new things; a stale mind and narrow view is boring to be around.
- Your life is shaped by what you 'feed' it, physically, emotionally and spiritually.
- Don't let anyone underestimate you but yourself. Think

positive, be confident and never doubt your abilities, values and confidence.

- Forget the illusion that happiness will arrive when you get that car, house, job or woman. True happiness is in the journey.
- Be respectful, honest, interested and polite and this will come back to you.
- Live in the moment and you may see further than you ever have.
- Always be kind; the Karma bus misses no one.
- As soon as you 'get' each of life's lessons, you get to move on. If you really get the lesson you pass and don't have to repeat the class.
- The greatest thing in the world a father can give his child is being there. Love, encourage, support and stay young with your kids.
- Never stop laughing or making other people laugh.
- Live with purpose. When you are on course, you are powerful. You may stumble but you will not fall.
- Good manners exude style and are never forgotten.
- To move forward you have to give back.
- Move your body, exercise your mind and respect both, you only have one of each.
- The reason we have two ears and one mouth is to listen more and talk less.
- Think it, live it, be it.
- Always pay your way; having the title 'cheap' is cheap.
- Be thankful for what you have, you'll end up having more.
- Know exactly how much alcohol you can drink without losing your temper, your dignity, your values, your wallet or your sexual performance.

Personal measurements

Clothing fit is the most important component to look one's best. Record your measurements below following the directions in Chapter 1 — Size Does Matter.

Shirts

Chest   _____   cm

Neck   _____   cm

Sleeve   _____   cm

Suits

Chest   _____   cm

Neck   _____   cm

Sleeve   _____   cm

Pants

Waist   _____   cm

Inside leg   _____   cm

Outside leg   _____   cm

Shoes

Length   _____   cm

Width   _____   cm

For more information or to book in for a personal consultation, please visit www.styleshift.com.au or contact Paul directly at info@styleshift.com.au.